CHASING MOLECULES

CHASING MOLECULES

Poisonous Products, Human Health, and the
Promise of Green Chemistry

Elizabeth Grossman

◯ **ISLAND**PRESS / Shearwater Books
Washington | Covelo | London

A Shearwater Book
Published by Island Press

Copyright © 2009 Elizabeth Grossman

All rights reserved under International and Pan-American Copyright Conventions. No part of this book may be reproduced in any form or by any means without permission in writing from the publisher: Island Press, 1718 Connecticut Ave., NW, Suite 300, Washington, DC 20009.

SHEARWATER BOOKS is a trademark of The Center for Resource Economics.

Library of Congress Cataloging-in-Publication data.

Grossman, Elizabeth, 1957–
  Chasing molecules : poisonous products, human health, and the promise of green chemistry / Elizabeth Grossman.
     p. cm.
  "A Shearwater Book."
  Includes bibliographical references and index.
  ISBN-13: 978-1-59726-370-2 (cloth : alk. paper)
  ISBN-10: 1-59726-370-2 (cloth : alk. paper) 1. Environmental toxicology—Popular works. 2. Environmental chemistry—Industrial applications—Popular works. 3. Consumer goods—Toxicology—Popular works. I. Title.
  RA1226.G76 2010
  615.9′02—dc22

                                                                    2009028279

British Cataloguing-in-Publication data available.

Printed on recycled, acid-free paper

Manufactured in the United States of America

10 9 8 7 6 5 4 3 2 1

For Jane and Olivia, with love and hope

In virtually every aspect in society, it has long been acknowledged that preventing a problem is superior to trying to solve it once it has been created.
—Paul Anastas and John Warner, 2000

Contents

Prologue

It is late September 2008 and I'm standing in the lobby of a Manila hotel where I'm attending a meeting about occupational health, safety, and environmental issues for workers throughout Asia. On a television screen nearby, polar bears are diving off a small ice floe. Later in the day, I visit the National Museum of the Philippines where we tour an exhibit of prize winners in a 2007 Filipino art competition. One of the paintings shows a woman clad in a dress constructed of images of cars and smokestacks. She has her hands over her eyes in a gesture of despair and is up to her hips in water. In this tropical island nation, merely 15 degrees north of the equator, where many people live on the water's edge, disappearing polar bear habitat—a sign of global warming and harbinger of rising sea levels—has local relevance. Over the next several days I meet people who work in factories that make clothing, electronics, machinery, and other products. When asked to name their top concerns about their working conditions, leading the list are the impacts of chemicals to reproductive health and the health of future generations. When asked what they would do to improve workplace safety, all say, "Remove the chemical hazard. Substitute something safer."

This is, in essence, the story this book explores. Over the past century our reliance on petroleum and coal has made available a vast quantity of hydrocarbons. These byproducts of fuel refining have become the foundation for the overwhelming majority of our synthetic materials—manufactured substances that go into everything from computers to cosmetics. We've managed to create tens of thousands of such new materials—substances that exist nowhere in nature—and these materials now permeate every aspect of our lives. They have made possible the creation of countless useful and often ingenious products: the lightweight, shatterproof, flame-resistant plastics used in electronics, aircraft, sports gear, and motor vehicles; waterproof coatings for textiles; flexible plastics that go into medical tubing and children's toys; nonstick surfaces for food packaging; thin films that enable microchip etching; and polymers delicate enough to coat an eyelash, to name but a few. It's hard to imagine life without them. These materials were designed to make life easier, more efficient, more convenient and, in many cases, safer. And many do.

But many of these substances also behave in ways that make them hazardous to human health and the environment. A number of these synthetic chemicals, scientists are discovering, are capable of interfering with the biological mechanisms that determine the health of any living organism. These materials, it turns out, have been changing the world's chemistry, in some instances altering the most fundamental building blocks of life on Earth. As a result, the entire chemistry of the planet—from the cellular level to entire ecosystems—is now different than at any other time in history.

This story is a sobering one. Yet what I learned while working on this book—and even more, the people I met—inspire me to think that the problems created by our past century's choice of materials are not insoluble. As with climate change, it's not possible to turn back the clock and erase all of the damage caused. However, if we build on the efforts now underway to create alternative materials that are safe for human health and the environment, and if we can prevent further pollution by existing harmful substances, great improvement and much recovery are possible. Where toxic contaminants have been taken out of use—through volun-

tary efforts or more often when regulations are established and en-
forced—affected populations and individuals, if sufficiently healthy and
resilient, can and often do recover. But we have to act swiftly. As Paul
Anastas, director of the Center for Green Chemistry and Green Engineering at Yale University and a founder of the green chemistry movement
has said succinctly, "We don't have a decade to blow."[1]

Since the 1950s, if not earlier, scientists have been aware of the acute
adverse incidental impacts of numerous petroleum-based synthetic pesticides and industrial chemicals—immediate severe reactions in some cases
(to the respiratory or nervous system, for example), severe disorders such
as cancer or birth defects in others. In the past several decades, however,
our knowledge of how these substances make their way into the environment and our bodies, and how these widely used synthetic chemicals can
affect healthy living cells, has grown remarkably. We now know that such
chemicals are migrating not only from industrial and waste sites but also
from finished products designed for everyday use, products that range
from furniture and textiles to electronics, toys, and personal care products. Many of these substances are mobile, made up of molecules that literally become detached from finished products and move into adjacent
air, water, soil, or onto other nearby surfaces. Many also have chemical
structures and elements that resist environmental degradation, enabling
some to persist for years and even decades. Many are traveling the global
environment with air and ocean currents. Many are also present in indoor
air and household dust. And many are now being found literally everywhere on Earth—often far, even continents away, from where they were
made, used, or disposed of—and in virtually everyone who's been tested.

In addition to their sometimes acute adverse health impacts, many
of these synthetic chemicals interact—often at very low levels of exposure—with vital biological mechanisms in ways that can result in health
problems that may not become apparent until years or even generations
later. Among these effects are reproductive, metabolic, immune system,
and neurological disorders—effects that can lead to such chronic conditions as diabetes, obesity, and learning difficulties. Many of these chemicals have been identified as endocrine disruptors for their ability to

interfere with the workings of the hormones that regulate and maintain a number of the body's reproductive, metabolic, and other vital systems. Overall, these compounds are so pervasive that nearly all babies in the United States are now born with synthetic chemicals already in their bloodstreams.

❖ ❖ ❖

A few years ago, research into local water quality issues where I live in Portland, Oregon, led me to investigate the environmental and health impacts of the high-technology industry, an investigation that led to publication of *High Tech Trash: Digital Devices, Hidden Toxics, and Human Health.* What I learned fascinated me and prompted wider questions about what scientists are learning about the behavior of many commonly used synthetic chemicals, particularly those that are being released by finished consumer products and making their way into the environment, our food, and our bodies. Why, I wondered, are flame retardants and chemicals used to make nonstick and water-resistant surfaces turning up in seals, sea turtles, and salmon as well as in ordinary supermarket foods including cheese, chicken, eggs, and microwave popcorn? I wanted to know why 95 percent of Americans tested by the Centers for Disease Control had chemicals used to make common plastics and cosmetics in their blood. Why virtually all the nursing mothers tested in the United States were passing these substances on to their babies. Why people who do not live near or work in industrial plants are testing positive for multiple synthetic chemicals, some of which have been off the market for more than thirty years. And why we couldn't design useful synthetic materials without properties that disrupt fundamental biological mechanisms and cause problems that persist, literally, for generations.

There are far more of these synthetic chemicals than could ever be described in a single book. I've chosen to focus on a number of these that are found in widely used materials, that were introduced for commercial use with the assumption that they were biologically inert, and that scientists now believe can cause serious adverse health and environmental effects. While some of these chemicals have been in use for many years, their environmental and health hazards—particularly their ability to disrupt endocrine hormone functions and other vital biological and genetic mechanisms—have only recently been recognized. Many of these chemicals are found in a vast number of globally distributed products, many of them in everyday use. This has resulted in what are effectively millions of point sources of pollution that are both widely dispersed and in close proximity to people. Altogether, this presents a very different prospect for controlling these hazards than does curbing releases from large stationary sources like factories or waste sites. Although we are also now all exposed to multiple chemicals, scientists have just begun to study the effects of these combined exposures. And although conditions on the factory floor and in farm fields have improved considerably in recent decades, workers worldwide continue to be exposed to hazardous chemicals on the job.

Use of many of the older generation of long-lasting synthetic chemicals Rachel Carson wrote about in *Silent Spring* has been restricted or banned in many places, but these pesticides, along with industrial fluids like PCBs, are actually still with us, as are many other industrial chemicals that have entered the environment over the past four decades or more. These substances are not biodegradable by ordinary processes, and some even resist breakdown through current wastewater treatment, and thus persist in groundwater, oceans, lakes, rivers, soil, ice, and snow. Many of these persistent pollutants, both the older and the more recently recognized contaminants, also have a chemistry that enables them to accumulate in fat cells and fat tissue, and thus—as contaminated plants and animals are eaten—to climb the food web. In some locations, warming temperatures are now accelerating the release of contaminants held in place by snowfields, sea ice, permafrost, and frozen soil and as a result are affecting animals—and people—already stressed by climate change.

Historically, regulations and safety standards aimed at protecting human and environmental health from chemical hazards have been designed to limit exposure to what's considered an acceptable level of risk—how much of a toxic substance one can be exposed to without it causing observable, measurable harm. In the early 1990s, a new approach to preventing chemical pollution began to be articulated by proponents of what's called "green chemistry," a subject that is central to the discussion in this book and a discipline that has the potential to transform the world of manufactured materials as well as how we consider a material's safety.

The fundamental tenet of green chemistry is that preventing a problem—eliminating hazards at the outset or the design stage—is superior to trying to contain or control it once the problem has occurred. Put simply, not sending noxious fumes out of a smokestack is preferable to trying to deal with that pollution once it's in the chimney, let alone drifting through the air. Similarly, if a detergent is formulated without persistent pollutants, we don't have to worry about what happens to the suds after they go down the drain. What successful green chemistry promises is the prevention of chemical pollution by designing materials that are inherently environmentally benign.

An elegantly simple approach, green chemistry actually represents a radical departure from how commercial synthetic chemistry has been practiced. It asks specific questions about synthetic compounds' environmental behavior and toxicity from the beginning of the design stage all the way through manufacture, use, and end-of-product-life—questions that typically have not been asked in detail until these materials are launched into commercial production. Answering these questions faithfully and accurately—and with the aim of continually improving product safety—is what gives green chemistry the potential to revolutionize our choice and use of manufactured materials. Green chemistry efforts are underway all around the world, and many successful products designed according to green chemistry principles are now in use. The science is still in its infancy, but the more we learn about the hazards of so many widely used synthetic chemicals, the more compelling green chemistry becomes.

❖ ❖ ❖

Adding considerably to the promise of green chemistry are the energetic and dynamic scientists who are leaders in the field. Engaging and eager to share their work, they bring a style of storytelling and sense of social purpose to their science that has the potential, I think, to be as transformative as the new materials they're out to create. Among those I was lucky enough to meet and whose work is part of the story told here is John Warner, one of green chemistry's founders and whose own story in many ways mirrors that of the growing concern about existing toxics and the need to do something about them.

"My mission," says John Warner over coffee in the living room of his house in Lowell, Massachusetts, on a sunny spring morning, "is to convince the next generation that this is the most important thing they can do." It may be no exaggeration to say that the mission Warner is on could change the world. He wants to put the next generation of chemists and chemical engineers to work on behalf of green chemistry, creating new materials that meet high technical and performance standards and that are environmentally benign. Spending time with beakers, test tubes, and molecular equations—no matter how novel—may not sound revolutionary, but what Warner advocates could effect a radical transformation not only of nearly every manufactured product we now use, but also of how we determine the safety of those products. A transition to green chemistry would also go a long way toward ending the recurring cycle of persistent, pervasive, and toxic pollution unleashed over the past century.

Making this transition will require a new approach to the design of new materials and products. It will almost certainly bring about a shift away from reliance on petrochemicals as the base for so many of our current synthetic materials, a move that is already—however gradually—underway. It will also require a new approach to how we assess the efficacy of new materials and their environmental effects. As Warner and his colleague Paul Anastas express it in their landmark text *Green Chemistry: Theory and Practice*, "Green chemistry involves the design and redesign of chemical syntheses and chemical products to prevent pollution and thereby solve environmental problems."[2]

Warner himself is a compact, animated, and energetic man in his forties. Apart from sartorial improvements, his appearance hasn't changed all that much since the 1980s college photos he's happy to share as he talks about how he became a chemist. He speaks with an infectious enthusiasm I had not associated with chemistry before I began work on this book. "I'm a synthetic organic chemist. I make molecules," says Warner with a touch of disarming self-deprecation. Discussions of lab benches and regulatory policies may limit the glamour factor, but Warner is something of a rock star in the world of green chemistry.

"Why do we have red dye that causes cancer, plasticizers that cause birth defects?" Warner asks rhetorically. "We're lucky if 10 percent of the stuff we use is benign," he tells me. "Sixty-five percent of what we have now, we don't know how to make safely."

What distinguishes green chemistry—as defined by Warner and Anastas—from chemistry as historically practiced is that green chemistry is intended to be "benign by design." Instead of dealing with the byproducts, waste products, and environmental and health impacts of a newly synthesized material *after* it's been made, green chemistry asks synthetic chemists, materials designers, and engineers to follow "a set of principles that reduces or eliminates the use or generation of hazardous substances in the design, manufacture," and use of chemical products—all problems that, historically, we've dealt with after the fact, most often after the substance is already in high-volume commercial production.[3]

Opting for less waste, fewer—or no—hazardous materials, greater materials and energy efficiency, and nontoxic end products sounds like a no-brainer. One would be hard-pressed to find disagreement with these goals. Considerably more contentious and difficult is refashioning our historical approach to chemical hazard and risk.

Read the history of any debate over the toxicity of a substance used in commercial products and you'll quickly see that the discussion focuses on "how toxic" a substance is and how much of the material in question one can be exposed to without harm. As Warner and Anastas note, the debate over how these environmental hazards should be gauged and how uncertainties about potential harm should be resolved has been ongoing for at least a generation and will likely continue for at least another. Given this situation, the scientific community has a choice, in their view: It can either allow itself to be paralyzed by uncertainty and "not attempt to address the concerns for human health and the environment" or it can accept the reality of these impacts and begin to reduce and eliminate them by adopting what I will describe as an ecological approach to materials design.[4]

"Green chemistry is not complicated although it is often elegant. It holds as its goal nothing less than perfection," write Anastas and Warner.[5] "When we reflect upon the issues confronting society today, we have to reflect upon the materials that are in the environment. In the history of humanity what better time is there to be a chemist, designing new materials?"[6] Warner says emphatically. These are grand ambitions but their mission is also personal. Their advocacy for green chemistry grows out of personal concerns and reflects the background and experience of both Warner and Anastas in the world of academic and industrial chemistry—and for Paul Anastas, in government—as well as in their family roots in New England communities long known for their mills and factories.

The day I visit Warner is his last as director of the University of Massachusetts–Lowell's Center for Green Chemistry. Warner had been teaching at UMass–Lowell for more than ten years and is resigning as professor of plastics engineering to establish the Warner Babcock Institute for Green Chemistry.

Lowell is a fitting place to see green chemistry in historical perspective. The city was long at the industrial heart of New England, a community that for more than 200 years has been home at one time or another to textile mills, tanneries, shoe factories, electronics, high technology and, yes, chemical manufacturing. This is a region long familiar with industrial and chemical pollution. The Warner Babcock Institute has its offices in Woburn, the town not far from Boston where, for years, the W. R. Grace Company had dumped industrial chemicals that were eventually linked to a cluster of local childhood leukemia cases, some fatal. The story and subsequent lawsuit against the company were made famous by Jonathan Harr's 1995 book, *A Civil Action*. Reducing chemical exposure on the job and in the community is very much a backyard issue here.

The predicament of pervasive synthetic chemical pollution has come about, Warner argues, in part because getting a PhD in chemistry in the United States today does not require a class in toxicology or environmental chemistry. "How can we ask people to go to work in industry and make safe products if they don't know how," asks Warner. As synthetic chemists—scientists who create new materials in the lab—"we don't even have a language to talk about safe materials."

Warner grew up not far from here, in Quincy, Massachusetts, just south of Boston—a city known for being home to John Adams and for its shipyards and granite quarries. "My mother had ten brothers and sisters, and I have thirty-five first cousins, and I grew up with them all nearby," Warner tells me, his voice rich with the round open vowels characteristic of the area. He is part of the first generation in his family to go to college and worked his way through school. Warner began his academic career not in science but as a music major and as a member of a band he and his buddies called the Elements. But as Warner tells me, his life changed direction after his close friend and bandmate, James O'Neil, died of leukemia in 1981. "It wasn't the same after that," Warner says of the band, and he switched his major to chemistry.

Warner recalls overhearing one of his professors at the University of Massachusetts talking about chemical research. "I was intrigued," says Warner, who turned out to be exceptionally talented as a synthetic chemist. "I think there's an innate instinct to create. Whether it's composing a piece of music or designing a molecule—they're the same thing neurologically. I can be a creative person and do science."

"I've synthesized over a hundred molecules that never existed before," Warner tells me. By the time he finished graduate school at Princeton in 1988, with a PhD in organic chemistry, Warner had published seventeen scientific papers—many on compounds related to pharmaceuticals, particularly anticancer drugs—a volume of research publication he immodestly but matter-of-factly says is "perhaps unprecedented."

One day Warner got a call from Polaroid offering him a job in their exploratory research division. So he went to work synthesizing new materials for the company, inventing compounds for photographic and film processes. Describing his industrial chemistry work in an article for the Royal Chemistry Society, Warner wrote: "I synthesized more and more new compounds. I put methyl groups and ethyl groups in places where they had never been. This was my pathway to success."[7] There was even a series of compounds he invented that, in his honor, became known as "Warner complexes."

Warner had married in graduate school and while working at Polaroid had three children. His youngest and second son, John—born in 1991—was born with a serious birth defect. It was a liver disease, Warner tells me, caused by the absence of a working billiary system (which creates the secretions necessary for digestion). Despite intensive medical care, surgery, and a liver transplant, John died in 1993 at age two. "You can't imagine what it was like," says Warner. "Laying awake at night, I started wondering if there was something I worked with, some chemical that could possibly have caused this birth defect," Warner recalls. He knows it's unlikely that this was the case, but contemplating this possibility made him acutely aware of how little attention he and his colleagues devoted to the toxicity or ecological impacts of the materials they were creating.

"I never had a class in toxicology or environmental hazards," Warner tells me and shows me a slide from a lecture he gives that reads from top to bottom in increasingly large type: "I have synthesized over 2,500 compounds! I have never been taught what makes a chemical toxic! I have no idea what makes a chemical an environmental hazard! I have synthesized over 2,500 compounds! *I have no idea what makes a chemical toxic!*" "We've been monkeys typing Shakespeare," he adds.

"The chemical synthesis toolbox is really full, and 90 percent of what's in that toolbox is really nasty stuff." It's a coincidence and reality of history, Warner tells me, but the petroleum industry has been the primary creator of materials for our society. "Most of our materials' feedstock is petroleum. As petroleum is running out, things will have to change." But, he says, it's an oversimplification to say that using naturally occurring, nonpetroleum materials will automatically be safe.

Industrial chemistry has historically relied on the criteria of performance and cost. But safety, Warner adds, has not been an equal part of the equation. Green chemistry puts safety as well as material and energy efficiency on a par with performance and cost. This sounds like common sense, but our economic system's overwhelming focus on performance—

combined with the past century's reliance on what have been inexpensive petroleum-based feedstocks (or base materials)—have created a vast number of high-performing but environmentally inefficient and detrimental materials.

What we need to do, says Warner, is link the design and function of new materials and new molecular synthesis with an assessment of their hazard and risk. "Historically, we've mitigated risk," explains Warner, "and we've done this by trying to limit exposure." If we eliminate hazard in the first place, the issue of quibbling over exposure limits—where all of our chemical pollutant regulatory energy has been focused—goes away. If you haven't created and put materials with inherent hazards into production and commercial uses, you do not have to decide, for example, if it's safe to expose high school but not elementary and middle school students to lead dust emanating from artificial turf, or wonder why New York allows its residents to be exposed to higher levels of a potentially carcinogenic indoor air contaminant than does California.

"We've taken it as a fait accompli that chemistry must be dangerous. But the cost of using hazardous materials is exponentially more costly," says Warner. "There is no reason that a molecule must be toxic in order to perform a particular task." The cost of storing, transporting, treating, and disposing of hazardous materials, not to mention the expense of liability, and corporate responsibility for worker health and safety, are among the high costs associated with using hazardous materials. Corporations have seldom been required to take responsibility for hazardous materials they used or produced—apart from product failures—beyond some aspects of the manufacturing stage. The costs of environmental impacts were not considered an explicit cost of doing business; they were what are referred to technically as externalities. As that view has slowly begun to change, with pressure from consumers, unions, government regulators, and the courts, manufacturers are increasingly motivated to find ways to reduce these costs. Green chemists argue that one of the most effective ways to do so is by designing more environmentally benign and efficient products.

"What you do in industrial chemistry," says Warner, "is make and break chemical bonds. And in nature weak molecular bonds—bonds that come together and apart again, that assemble and reassemble, and are reversible—dominate." This is important, he tells me, because "if we can learn what molecules 'want' to do—if we can learn what they do in nature—we should be able to make better, less toxic products." If we can do that, we won't be fighting nature or introducing ultimately unwanted, often hazardous, and inefficient elements into the synthetic process.

✢ ✢ ✢

It was on a trip to Washington, D.C., in the early 1990s to try and secure Environmental Protection Agency approval for some new materials he'd synthesized at Polaroid that Warner found himself in a conversation with Paul Anastas at the White House's Office of Science and Technology Policy. While working in the EPA's Office of Pollution Prevention and Toxics, Anastas had launched a program that provided grant money for research and development of new materials whose synthesis incorporated pollution prevention.[8]

Warner and Anastas quickly discovered they had much in common. Both were from the Boston area, both had studied chemistry as undergraduates at the University of Massachusetts, and during college Warner had played in a band with Anastas's brother Rick. Warner shows me a photo of their band, called A Touch of Brass, with the musicians sporting big collared black shirts and classic 1980s big hair. Fueled by shared background and interests, Anastas and Warner began talking about the need to create a science that would intentionally focus on waste and pollution prevention. Thus began their green chemistry collaboration.

With support from the Clinton administration's "Reinventing Government" initiative, Anastas persuaded the EPA to establish its Green Chemistry program. Anastas and Warner also helped launch what's called the Presidential Green Chemistry Challenge Award, a program that, since 1996, has recognized leading innovations in environmentally benign and pollution prevention chemistry. Many of these projects are strikingly collaborative, often involving university students and professors along with industry chemists and engineers. Every time a win-ner was announced at the awards ceremony I attended in 2007 an entire audience row of the

National Academy of Sciences auditorium stood up and walked onstage to claim the award to the clicking of family members' cameras. "The recipients of the Presidential Green Chemistry Challenge Award alone have eliminated enough hazardous substances to fill a train eight miles long," says Anastas.

These conversations with Anastas and others helped give Warner's career its present direction. "I had a great relationship with Polaroid," recalls Warner. "But after my son died, I left because I wanted to create the world's first green chemistry PhD program"—which he did, at the University of Massachusetts–Lowell in 2002.

Although green chemistry ideas have been out in the world as articulated by Warner, Anastas, and their colleagues for some years now, they have made few substantial inroads in standard academic science curricula in the United States. This means that, with few exceptions, we're still educating chemists to work without an ecological context. "I teach 'Chemistry for Poets,'" Warner tells me. "Chemistry for nonscientists is all about the environment, but the American Chemical Society that accredits U.S. academic chemistry programs includes no environmental studies in its requirements." India, on the other hand, has mandated that all universities have a year of green chemistry.

"Currently the green [chemistry] toolbox is rather empty," Warner says, referring to a repertoire of chemical combinations that can be drawn upon to create environmentally benign materials. "We're starting to fill that toolbox," but there's an urgent need for new materials. "I feel we need a factor of ten more people to go into science and chemistry. We don't have the solutions and we need to have them," says Warner. But, he says, "we need product performance. People don't want lousy products, and products won't succeed just because they're environmentally acceptable. People who are not on the front lines don't understand how difficult innovation is."

The most basic principle of green chemistry—that of eliminating hazard at the design stage—is quite persuasive to chemical manufacturers and industries that use these materials, as it can keep them ahead of the regulatory curve. Doing so saves the very costly process of reformulating an existing product line to meet new regulations or, worse, the need to recall a product. Eliminating hazard at the design stage also eliminates the torturous and prolonged negotiations over acceptable risk and exposure limits on which our current chemical regulations are based. Hang around discussions and conferences about U.S. chemical regulation and you'll quickly be shown a hockey-stick-shaped graph plotting the proliferation of American environmental legislation over the past century. Its upward slope begins gradually in the 1870s and begins to rise notably in the mid-1950s, then accelerates steeply in the 1960s and 1970s, climbing steadily into the mid-1990s. While enormous progress in environmental protection has been achieved in some areas, simply increasing the number of such regulations at either the federal or state level has clearly not proven to be the most effective way of preventing the proliferation of persistent and pervasive pollutants.

"I think we're at a tipping point," Warner says of green chemistry. "Corporate America is being pressured to have sustainability goals. With industry doing this, academia will have to come along." "We can be apolitical about this," notes Warner. "A molecule is not a Democrat or Republican, liberal or conservative. Industry is slowly coming along. Is the movement real or on paper? We can't measure intent, we can only look at behavior," he remarks.

"An absence of the narrative of hazard leads to industrial hazard," Warner tells me, emphasizing how important environmental and social context are to scientific invention. "Science trains people to suppress the narrative," he says—to work as if considerations of culture and history and language are entirely separate from science. "Our society has messed up by creating a situation where it's art versus science. But if we are part of the narrative, who would want to make a hazardous material? We need to bring the narrative back to science."

And ultimately? "We need to put the concept of 'green' chemistry out of business," Warner tells me. "It should just be chemistry. Green chemistry is just intelligent product design."

✤ ✤ ✤

Work on this book has made me aware of our material surroundings in a whole new way. Tracking molecules, unraveling the mysteries of their affinities and dynamics, and how they behave under different environmental conditions seems to me almost a form of anthropology or archaeology, so complex, interwoven, interdependent, and ever-evolving are their relationships. While often painstaking, this work is tremendously exciting. Identifying chemicals in a cloud plume, in a chunk of sea ice, vial of water, soil sample, slice of fish, or scoop of household dust yields clues to understanding both the health of the planet and each of us as individuals.

Scientists are professionally cautious and generally shy away from sweeping, dramatic statements. So I was surprised by the frankness and bold pronouncements so many are now making about the state of the world. This speaks, I think, to the urgency of redesigning our material future. We spent the twentieth century building economies and societies based around the power of petroleum and fossil fuels. The benefits have been enormous. Better living has been achieved through chemistry but it's now apparent that we need to do even better. As I'm writing this, the world is in economic turmoil and thinking about safer, cleaner materials may seem like a luxury. But based on what I've learned in the course of researching this book, these are changes we can not afford to do without.

CHAPTER ONE

There's Something in the Air

Clouds are building slowly along the horizon as afternoon breezes begin to stir the air. Cumulous clouds float over the northern shore of Lake Erie, casting shadows on fields of wheat and corn and soybeans. They float over the Tomato Capital of Canada. Over cattails and water lilies and disappearing bullfrogs. The breezes travel south over Lake Huron and over Ojibwe homelands on the south shore of the lake. They travel over the smokestacks of Sarnia, Detroit, and Windsor, and mix with air blowing north from Cleveland and the Ohio Valley. They ruffle flags on the small docks of homes along the St. Clair River, bending the plume of power-plant smoke and black-tipped flares from the refineries that shadow their backyards. They whip up waves at the mouth of the Detroit River and rock the fishing boats moored at the Wheatley Harbor where children scamper along the pier, casting lines in practice for the upcoming fishing derby.

It is because this Great Lakes region has the worst air quality and the highest ozone levels along the U.S.-Canadian border that I am standing in an Ontario bean field on a sweltering July day in 2007 with scientists who have set up mobile labs to map and measure what's in the air. It's here that airborne effluent from petrochemical and automotive factories, oil

1

refineries, and coal-fired power plants in Sarnia, about an hour's drive north of here, and factories in Windsor and Detroit along the U.S.-Canadian border, mixes with diesel exhaust from one of North America's busiest trucking corridors, which runs between Midwestern and Eastern industrial hubs. As air swirls above the Great Lakes, propelled by cool lake waters and heat from the sun, chemical reactions are taking place. Hydrocarbons, carbon monoxide and dioxide, nitrogen, sulfur, and persistent pollutants bounce around the troposphere.

Some of these chemicals will linger locally, as smog and particulates that will make some residents of this Great Lakes region wheeze and cause the blood vessels of others to constrict. Some will act as greenhouse gases and contribute to the climate-disrupting effects of global warming. Some will turn up in Great Lakes fish, for which the U.S. Environmental Protection Agency currently maintains some thirty-nine different chemical advisories.[1] Atop a buoy bobbing on the waves of Lake Erie, the scientists I'm visiting have placed a filter to catch pollutants that drift out over the water. Overhead, a small plane loaded with gear to monitor what's floating up near the clouds cruises over the farm fields, its buzz mingling with summer insect drone and distant traffic hum.

Later I'll drive through neighborhoods surrounding the factories that turn fossil fuel into the ingredients of plastics; solvents; fertilizers; pesticides; lubricants; synthetic fibers; surfactants; pharmaceuticals; moisture, stain, and flame repellants; cosmetics; and household cleaning and personal care products. Families in these neighborhoods carry the chemical constituents of these products in their bloodstreams.[2] Hospitalization rates in their communities are significantly higher than elsewhere in Canada as are rates of respiratory and cardiovascular disease. People who live here also have notably higher incidences of certain cancers—Hodgkin's disease and leukemia—than do other Ontario residents.[3] It's becoming increasingly clear that these illnesses are related to the thousands of tons of airborne pollutants that circulate through these communities. These chemicals may also impact residents' health in far less overt or acute ways, prompting subtle but significant changes in how genetic receptors and hormones behave and setting the stage for dysfunction that may take years or even generations to become apparent.

Some of these chemicals will also move on, mingling with soot, vehicle and agricultural emissions, and vented indoor air. They will travel on city breezes, with global air and water currents—with clouds, rain, snowmelt, pollen, oceans, rivers, and fog. Some will end up continents away from their points of origin, leapfrogging with seasonal weather patterns across county, state, and national borders. As a result of such chemical migrations, even the most remote and visually pristine places on Earth—high-altitude rain forests, coral reefs, and Arctic communities among them—are suffering the impacts of industrial pollution.

Later that same July, on a day when the sun barely set, in an Alaskan island village built on permafrost, I listened to residents express frustration, anxiety, and anger over not knowing how these kinds of lingering pollutants might be affecting their health and that of the animals they depend on for food. Some of the same chemicals wafting over those Ontario farm fields and found in the tissue of Great Lakes fish will be in ice samples I helped scientists bag a few months later, in December on the frozen Beaufort Sea. Tracking the journey of such pollutants further the following April, I watched gulls fly over water dotted with small ice floes off the north coast of the Norwegian islands of Svalbard, just 10 latitude degrees south of the North Pole. Brominated flame retardants—synthetic chemicals commonly used in upholstery and electronics—have been found in these birds and their eggs.

What makes this far-flung pollution perplexing is that while some of it comes from smokestacks, drainpipes, tail pipes, waste sites, and other industrial sources, many of these contaminants can be traced to and migrate out of products we use every day and seldom think could be the source of airborne or aquatic contamination. Our kitchens, offices, bathrooms, hospitals, and children's toy boxes are filled with these products. We clean our homes, clothes, and bodies with them. Travel in a car, airplane, or modern train and you are surrounded by them. Much of our food is grown, processed with, and affected by such chemicals. Agricultural, industrial, and urban runoff, along with what we flush down our own household drains, has filled our waterways with so many of these chemicals that they are now common in coastal environments. We wear them, eat them, and touch them constantly. Vacuum cleaner and drier lint are full of them. One scientist has recently posited that young children's exposure to such compounds may be proportionally higher than adults' because they touch hands to mouth so much more frequently and are in closer proximity to household dust.[4]

Many of these fugitive chemicals have turned out to be long-distance travelers that resist degradation in the environment. They are accumulating in groundwater, soil, aquatic sediment, glacial snow, and polar ice. Many last for years, even decades. Others, such as those that make up polycarbonate and polyvinyl chloride (PVC) plastics, migrate only short distances and do not last for extended periods of time but are nevertheless pervasive and so widely used as to be virtually inescapable in twenty-first-century, consumer-product-filled society.

Both the persistent pollutants and the less long-lasting but pervasive synthetic chemicals are turning up repeatedly in animals, plants, food, and in people, including those who do not work with these substances nor live anywhere near where chemical product manufacturing takes place. Though used commercially with the assumption that they are safe, a growing body of scientific evidence indicates many of these materials may in fact not be. While not acutely toxic at levels routinely encountered, it appears that even at low levels some of these compounds can disrupt normal cell function with a number of disturbing outcomes. Among these impacts is interference with endocrine system hormones and genetic mechanisms that regulate reproductive and neurological development and metabolism. Some are being linked to the recent rise in obesity and other metabolic disorders, including diabetes. Others are confirmed or suspected carcinogens, while some have been documented to both interfere with hormone function in ways that can result in early puberty and irregular reproductive cycles and promote certain cancers as well as interfere with chemotherapy drugs.[5] Adverse impacts are now being seen not only in laboratory experiments but also in field observations.

A number of these engineered materials have molecular structures that make them soluble in fat. If traveling with air or water and taken up by an animals or plants, these substances will lodge in, and over time can build up in, the fat cells of plant or animal tissue. As contaminated plants and animals are eaten so are these fat-soluble compounds, and thus they work their way up the food web. Polar bears, top predators with great stores of fat, have among the highest recorded levels of such chemicals. Residents of the Arctic, whose diet centers on marine mammals and fatty fish, have some of the highest levels of exposure to these toxics. Recent scientific investigations indicate that fat cells themselves can become reservoirs of these fat-soluble or lipophilic (fat loving) toxics, setting the stage for prolonged contact even when the external sources of exposure are removed.

Some of these chemicals—both the persistent and the shorter-lived pervasive compounds—have become so ubiquitous that they are now found in the vast majority of Americans tested for them.[6] Similar results have been found in such testing (known as biomonitoring) done all around the world, with nearly everyone's results revealing evidence of chemicals to which they have had no occupational or other previously recognized exposure. Flame retardants, plasticizers, and surfactants (synthetic chemicals that give soaps, detergents, lotions, paints, and inks, for example, their special textures and consistency) are being found in newborns' umbilical cord blood. An expert in this field has told me that no babies are born in this country today without at least some of these synthetics percolating through their bodies.[7]

These chemicals—compounds designed in laboratories and that exist nowhere in nature—have given us lightweight, durable, flexible, and waterproof materials. These synthetic materials can be manipulated to deliver medicine, help increase crop yields, and create the nerve centers of digital information systems. They have transformed our lives in countless efficacious ways and it's now hard to imagine life without them. Yet the chemistry of a great many of these synthetics is also changing the world in ways that extend far beyond their intended design. In some cases these materials have permanently altered the behavior of hormones that control metabolism and reproduction resulting in adverse health effects that are already showing up in wildlife and human populations.

Many of these compounds are so different from the products of natural chemistry, says one scientist, that "it is as if they dropped in from an alien world."[8] Another—John Warner—commented, "We're lucky if 10 percent of the chemicals we use are truly benign."[9] These manufactured chemicals are subtly changing environmental chemistry worldwide—the fundamental building blocks of life on Earth—on both a cellular and landscape scale. So many of these changes have already taken place that according to marine scientists studying the impact of these chemicals, "During the course of the last century, the planet has become and is now chemically different from any previous time."[10]

❖ ❖ ❖

Virtually everything on Earth is made up of chemicals, as any number of people who work for chemical manufacturing companies have pointed out to me. Chemicals are simply the elemental molecules that make up life on Earth. I've also been reminded that at certain doses, under certain circumstances, even the most environmentally benign substances (water is the oft-cited example) can be toxic. There are also natural sources of many hazardous materials—mercury, for example, or poisonous plants— so industry is not the sole source of environmental toxics. All this is certainly true. The chemicals I'm following in this book, however, are all deliberately manufactured or the result of environmental breakdown and recombination of commercially synthesized materials. None would be present in our lives if they had not been invented in a laboratory, and their hazard or toxicity is directly related to their molecular composition and design. Unlike an overdose of water, exposure to these synthetic chemicals is occurring under normal circumstances—not accidentally or as a result of any product misuse, although occupational exposure to some of these synthetics can cause serious problems—often over extended periods of time, and most often without warning signs of unusual odor, taste, or other immediate sensory distress signals.

We've been living with warnings about industrially synthesized and dispersed chemicals for decades now. But we've responded to these concerns on a piecemeal, substance-by-substance basis, taking one material off the market when its adverse effects have been recognized and substituting another without altering the framework of this process. This approach has discontinued use of some blatantly dangerous chemicals, and some scientists feel this has successfully reduced our exposure to the most hazardous toxics. But this approach has also allowed the commercial production of tens of thousands of new materials, many of which have turned out to be environmentally problematic, while allowing continued use of older known hazards either at low volumes or in places with less stringent environmental regulations. If evidence of chemical contamination were reported graphically on a global map, that chart would now be so riddled with blots that virtually no part of the world would be untouched.

Living with pollution and potentially hazardous materials is not new. Humans have been polluting ever since we began burning, mining, forging, milling, tanning, and dying. What is new in historical terms is the existence of so many synthetic chemicals—many of which are toxic—and the large number of such substances we are exposed to, often since before birth, and how impossible they are to avoid. We've now gotten a grip on some of the most egregious offenders in terms of large volumes of acutely toxic or noxious emissions—we're no longer using most ozone-depleting chemicals or spraying DDT across North America, for example—but the legacy of many of these substances is still with us and large quantities of hazardous effluent continue to flow from industrial point sources.

Some of the discontinued toxics, for example, PCBs (polychlorinated biphenyls)—which were used as industrial insulators and coolants, primarily in electrical equipment—are so persistent in the environment that although they were taken off the U.S. market in 1977 due to their carcinogenicity, they continue to be found almost everywhere scientists have looked. You "can't go anywhere on earth and not find PCBs," says John Stegeman, a senior scientist at the Woods Hole Oceanographic Institution who specializes in marine contaminants.[11] DDT was also taken out of use in the 1970s in the United States and Europe, but its chemical breakdown products continue to be found in people without current direct exposures in both North America and Europe. These are but two examples of such chemical persistence.

Environmental regulations enacted at about the same time as these product bans have effectively put the brakes on uncontrolled industrial emissions. But while we've worked hard to control these large fixed sources of chemical contamination, thanks to the global marketplace and supply chains of the twenty-first and late twentieth centuries, what we've added to this ongoing burden are potentially millions of new point sources of pollution—millions of individual products, mass-produced and launched at high volume and rapid pace into the world market— whose chemical contents permeate our lives and the world's environment. What is also new is that these chemicals are abroad in the world at a time when other crucial ecological dynamics are changing. These substances are interacting with biological mechanisms, individuals, species, and ecosystems that are also now affected by the impacts of global warming, natural resource depletion, and habitat destruction—all of which make us and the rest of nature more vulnerable than ever and which increase the urgency of finding solutions to this chemical pollution.

❖ ❖ ❖

Our overall use of synthetic chemicals is enormous. Every day, the United States alone uses or imports about 42 million pounds of such compounds.[12] Nearly 82,000 of these chemicals are registered for commerce in the United States. (The European Union, Canada, Japan, and other countries maintain comparable lists.) About 10 percent of these registered chemicals are produced or imported to the United States at volumes of 10,000 pounds or more each year. About 3,000 are produced or imported at quantities of 1 million or more pounds per year.[13] This list, administered by the U.S. Environmental Protection Agency, is only a partial accounting of all the chemicals in use, however. It does not include compounds like PCBs that are present in the environment but not in active use. Nor does it include chemicals like dioxins or the carbon dioxide, nitrogen, and sulfur oxides released in tailpipe emissions, substances that are breakdown or reaction products rather than deliberately manufactured materials.

Of the synthetic chemicals we're now using, about 90 percent are petrochemicals, a proportion that has grown to be about eighty times greater than it was some thirty years ago.[14] Using hydrocarbons as the building blocks for synthetic materials sets the stage for hazard: The basic physical properties of hydrocarbons (benzene, for example) make them toxic to many vital bodily systems. Hydrocarbons tend to evaporate easily, many are not water-soluble, and some have a viscosity that enhances their biological toxicity while others have what are called side-chains of chemicals that enable them to interact in often adverse ways with specific cellular mechanisms. At the same time, our reliance on petrochemicals reinforces our reliance on fossil fuel energy sources, adding to the practical challenges of shifting away from the materials driving climate change.

When it comes to keeping track of how these substances behave in the environment, of the 30,000 or so chemicals currently in common commercial use, the environmental and health impacts of only about 4 percent are routinely monitored. Some 75 percent have not been studied for such impacts at all.[15] Meanwhile, newly synthesized chemicals—which now include the products of nanotechnology (nanomaterials), infinitesimally small molecules that represent a whole new class of substances with novel properties and behaviors and barely studied toxicity—are put into commercial production at the rate of about 2,000 new chemicals every year. Altogether, over the past century, tens of thousands of synthetic chemicals have been released into the world's atmosphere.

In the United States and many other places in the world, new generations of synthetic chemicals were launched into commercial production—including at high volume—with little or no knowledge of their long-term impacts on human health and the environment. In the United States, even when seriously adverse effects of chemicals have been detected and confirmed, many toxic chemicals—including the suspected human carcinogens formaldehyde and trichloroethylene, for example—have remained in production or in use in products sold in the country for years. And our system of chemical regulation, which is based on reducing exposure only after a chemical has been shown to be harmful, has made it

extremely slow and cumbersome to effectively take a hazardous substance out of circulation or to establish effective protective national safety
standards.

The increasingly recognized dangers of such chemicals have prompted
both a move toward new types of regulations and greater efforts to develop alternative materials through green chemistry. In December 2006
the European Union passed legislation establishing a chemical management policy known as REACH—Registration, Evaluation, and Authorization of Chemicals. In contrast to most existing chemical regulation—
particularly in the United States—REACH requires chemical manufacturers to disclose health and safety information about their products (for
new products this must happen before they're marketed commercially)
and replace the most hazardous chemicals with safer substitutes when
available. Effective as of June 2007, REACH applies to all chemicals sold
in the EU, including those made by U.S. companies and others outside of
Europe. Similar legislation has been passed in Canada and Japan. Although
the Bush administration initially lobbied vigorously against REACH, U.S.
legislation called the "Kid Safe Chemical Act" that works similarly but is
limited to chemicals used in products designed for infants and children,
was introduced in May 2008 by the House and Senate. The bill failed to
pass, but it or similar legislation may be reintroduced. While it's too soon
to know the results of REACH or any comparable regulations, increasing
consumer awareness is prompting changes as well.

As I write, a groundswell of public concern over the health impacts of
chemicals that compose polycarbonate and polyvinyl chloride plastics is
pushing manufacturers and retailers of baby bottles, pacifiers, toddlers'
sippy cups, other children's products, and refillable water bottles to
switch to alternative materials. Europe and Canada are already phasing
out some of these chemicals starting with products designed for infants
and children. Beginning in 2009, a bill signed into law in August 2008
bars half a dozen PVC plasticizers from children's products. More than a
dozen U.S. states have introduced bills to bar bisphenol A, the polycarbonate chemical building block, from children's products—but as of May
2009, only two such bans have passed, one in Minnesota and the other in

Chicago. Meanwhile, European legislation restricting certain synthetic chemicals with known adverse health impacts has prompted numerous manufacturers to redesign or reformulate products ranging from nail polish to IV tubes to computers.

Given the history of these chemical products, rules that protect proprietary information (the secret formulas for these substances), and absence of independent third-party oversight, how are we to be assured of any new material's safety, now, ten, or twenty or more years from now? This is where John Warner and his green chemistry colleagues come in.

It's unlikely that we will return to making everything out of metal, stone, glass, and wood or that we'll abandon all synthetic fibers and pharmaceuticals. So the question at the heart of green chemistry is how to design molecules and materials that will perform desired tasks without adverse impacts—ideally a material that is resource-efficient and environmentally benign at every stage of a product's life. As two of the world's leading proponents of green chemistry—and in many ways its founders—John Warner and Paul Anastas, director of the Center for Green Chemistry and Green Engineering at Yale University, explain, "Green chemistry involves the design and redesign of chemical syntheses and chemical products to prevent pollution and thereby solve environmental problems."[16]

Work in the green chemistry field has really only gotten underway within the past decade or so—but new nontoxic chemicals designed to replace existing problematic synthetics are already in use. One striking example is Columbia Forest Products' formaldehyde-free plywood and particle board that uses a nontoxic adhesive developed to mimic the substance mollusks use to cling to rocks. Another is SC Johnson's reformulation of its stretchy plastic Saran food wrap to eliminate polyvinylidene chloride, a synthetic that includes carcinogenic chemical components and waste products. Other green chemicals are being developed as environmental cleaning agents that detoxify persistent pollutants already in the environment. Manufacturers and retailers as well as large-volume purchasers are involved in these product-shifting efforts—companies that include cleaning-product companies such as Clorox and Sysco Systems, pharmaceutical giants Pfizer and Schering-Plough, specialty chemical producer Rohm and Haas, agribusiness conglomerate Archer Daniels Midland, and others including Nike, Ikea, International Paper, Wal-Mart, and the U.S. Army, to name a few.

As large companies move away from known chemicals of concern and devise new strategies, they are discovering that, contrary to common perception, such innovations do not necessarily add to the overall cost of business. Some—InterfaceFLOR, the world's largest manufacturer of modular carpet, for example—have increased market share by adopting environmentally friendly practices and products. Other companies, pharmaceutical manufacturers among them, are attracted to the prospect of green chemistry for the savings it can bring through resource efficiency and reduced costs associated with the entire production process.

That said, the benign synthetics now in use represent but a small fraction of the shift that could take place both in terms of products and processes. There are also varying interpretations of what makes a chemical product green, and any number of apparent contradictions in existing product lines and processes. Green chemistry is not a magic wand, but what is happening is real and already far from a fringe movement or boutique trend.

Yet perhaps even more fundamental to green chemistry than the idea of substituting a benign material for one that is hazardous, is its departure from the historical approach to designing new materials and to commercial chemical production, which has focused overwhelmingly on performance and price. Green chemistry advocates are quick to say that their products must perform at least as well or better than existing, less environmentally benign materials. They also quickly add that to be commercially viable, these new products must end up on the net profit side of the balance sheet. But what's historically been absent from the calculus of commercial chemical production—or that of other manufactured products for that matter—is a full accounting for the cost of environmental impacts, short- or long-term. Green chemists recognize that these costs must be addressed.

Assessing a product's environmental impacts is not as clear-cut as it might seem. To begin, the outlines of the product's footprint must be defined—parameters for which there are not yet common standards. This may sound arcane but setting these boundaries is essential to capturing an accurate picture of a product's impacts, as deciding how far up the materials stream to go and which resources to include will produce widely varying results.

Listen to discussions of environmental impact and product life and you'll likely hear the phrases "life-cycle analysis," "cradle-to-cradle," "cradle-to-grave," and "cradle-to-gate." All can be variously and subjectively defined. A life-cycle analysis is generally understood to analyze and account for the environmental impacts of a product's entire manufacturing process, its impacts while in use, and its impacts when the product is no longer useful. Cradle-to-cradle assumes the premise of a closed production and product life-cycle loop—in which materials are reclaimed and reused, while cradle-to-grave assumes disposal rather than reuse or recycling for at least some portion of the product when it's discarded. Cradle-to-gate, meanwhile, has cropped up as a way for companies to measure the environmental footprint of their products but to stop at the factory gate—excluding what happens when that product goes out into the world. The proliferation of terms indicates that assessing environmental impacts is far from a standardized process and is often more of an afterthought than an integral consideration from the beginning of the manufacturing process for synthetic chemicals or any other product.

One of the astonishing things I learned while talking to green chemistry advocates and chemical engineers—and that helps explain why there has been so little attention to anything like footprint analysis—is that neither toxicology nor ecology has been required as part of a chemist's academic training. Historically, during the design phase, chemists work feverishly to get the next best material on the market before their competitors. Questions about the health, safety, and environmental impacts of their inventions typically came later. Safety testing and documentation is required for chemicals going into commercial production, but

protocols and questions that would detect the kind of chemical migration and the biological impacts we're now seeing on a global scale have
generally been absent from this evaluation process. Advocates of green
chemistry aim to change this, too.

Green chemistry is not a set of easy answers or an instant solution.
But it has the potential to completely change the nature of our synthetic
materials. Neither a brand nor a prescriptive labeling program, green
chemistry is a philosophy outlined by a set of principles that, if followed,
will create profoundly safer, more environmentally benign materials than
most we now use.[17] These materials will be made efficiently and result in
products without the persistence, byproducts, and costly waste issues that
are responsible for so many of the problems that plague industrial chemistry as it's traditionally been practiced. Paul Anastas and John Warner
call it a "revolutionary philosophy" for the way it upends the historical approach to chemical safety.

Instead of simply opening the universal kitchen cabinet of chemical
ingredients and choosing whatever will create a material with the desired
performance (ideally as quickly and cheaply as possible) then waiting for
someone else to test safety later on, proponents of green chemistry ask
synthetic chemists to assess safety and to avoid hazard at every step of design and synthesis. Are the basic materials toxic? Are the ingredients that
facilitate chemical reactions and bonding hazardous? Are dangerous
waste products created during synthesis? Are the required reactions and
production process resource-efficient? Will the final product be hazardous in any way during use or disposal? These are among the questions
green chemistry asks, not after a new material has been synthesized but
as it is being designed.

We have behind us a century or more of chemical products based on
syntheses that often rely on highly hazardous materials—phosgene, for
example, a highly toxic chlorine compound known as a nerve gas during
World War I, is used in the process of making many common synthetics
including plastics, upholstery foams, and synthetic fibers. In contrast,
green chemistry entails creating what amounts to a new alphabet and

grammar of chemical synthesis. As Amy Cannon, another leading green chemist, readily points out, green chemistry may sound fuzzy and soft—particularly now that the word "green" is slapped on everything from packages of toilet paper to motor oil, lipstick, and shoes—but, she says, it's actually much harder to practice, and it requires more analytical steps than conventional chemistry.

Green chemistry is also revolutionary in that it operates from a foundation that runs contrary to the basis of several generations' worth of policies regulating chemical safety. These policies have removed some egregiously bad chemical actors from the scene but have also prolonged the use of countless other hazardous materials, resulting in the environmental release of vast quantities of pollutants and the exposure of millions of people to substances with the distinct potential to harm human health. By focusing safety efforts on controlling risk, we've accepted the presence in our lives of numerous chemical hazards, from long-recognized toxins like lead to volatile organic compounds like trichloroethylene and perchlorate, to more recently recognized endocrine disruptors. This approach has also resulted in the confusing situation of having different levels of exposure to the same substance deemed acceptable in different geographic locations. Why should babies in Canada receive one kind of protection and American babies another? Why are women in Europe protected from chemical exposures that women in the United States are not, while residents of California receive more stringent protection than New Yorkers? "We have to turn the aircraft carrier around," says Terry Collins, who directs the Institute for Green Science at Carnegie Mellon University, "and get the hazard out."

Such efforts are underway all around world and, as noted, are being undertaken by some of the world's largest chemical companies and manufacturers. The proportion of currently available synthetic materials that are wholly products of green chemistry as yet represents but a small fraction of those now in use. But the impetus to explore environmentally benign alternatives to widely used problematic synthetics is growing. Altering manufacturing processes to eliminate hazardous and copious waste products, and to eliminate the need for hazardous process chemicals, may ultimately reduce production costs significantly because handling and disposing of toxic materials is expensive.

While some of the pressure to eliminate hazardous materials stems from manufacturers' desire to reduce production costs—including those of complying with regulations—there is also incentive to meet the growing consumer interest in safer products, whether it's baby bottles, mattresses, laptops, or makeup. When this interest is accompanied by regulation of recognized chemical hazards—or even the prospect of such regulation—design of more environmentally benign products accelerates. We've seen this already begin to happen with consumer electronics, cosmetics, textiles, and toys.

Among the notable changes of the past decade or so is how much more quickly the general public can access information on potential product hazards—and the speed with which the information is shared. Thanks to the Internet and e-mail, scientific studies, reports, and news bulletins make their way to far more offices and households around the globe than ever before, resulting in greater consumer awareness and, often, heightened concern. Concern from the public and from scientists has pushed policy makers—particularly in Europe but also in the United States—toward consideration and implementation of legislation, such as REACH, that takes a more precautionary approach to chemical use. It has also increased demand from consumers—institutional, corporate, and individual—for products without adverse health or environmental impacts.

❖ ❖ ❖

Scientists are professionally cautious. Their day-to-day work—in the field and in the lab—focuses on what is effectively one jigsaw puzzle piece at a time. Years of data collection and analysis are involved in creating each puzzle piece before it's ready to be snapped into place, and still more before any panoramic picture takes shape. But in the past year, while working on this book, I've heard impressively credentialed scientists make emphatic statements about the state of the world that astounded me for the depth and breadth of their concern.

"If we wait for comparable human data and it comes out like animal data, we aren't going to be breeding as a species," I was told by Patricia Hunt, Meyer Distinguished Professor at Washington State University's School of Molecular Biosciences. "Based on what we know now, why wait to count the numbers and the adverse events. Why wait until it's too late?" said Grace Egeland, Canada Research Chair in Environment, Nutrition, and Health at McGill University. "We're at a crossroads in the choices we make today as a civilization between a bad or a really bad future," Dave Barber, Canada Research Chair in Arctic System Science at the University of Manitoba, told me.

Our manipulation of natural elements has, undeniably, improved the quality of life in innumerable ways. Yet it now seems abundantly clear that our interference with Earth's natural environmental chemistry has thrown ecological systems—large and small—seriously out of balance. And the sources of what's forcing global climate change, it turns out, coincide with those of the materials responsible for changing environmental chemistry. The chemical emissions prompting the climatic changes we're now seeing have largely the same petrochemical origins as the synthetic chemicals altering essential cellular behavior in plants and animals, including humans, worldwide. The materials prompting global warming and all of its climate-disrupting impacts are thus, in effect, the backstory to that of these problematic mobile chemical contaminants that are interfering with the cellular and genetic processes vital to health.

We are in this fix largely because, over the course of the past century, worldwide we became a petrochemical society. It seems clear that solutions to our current dilemma will ultimately lie in our ability to move away from overwhelming reliance on fossil fuels, at least in the way we use them now. Aside from refashioning our main sources of energy, a large part of that shift away from petrochemicals will entail not only designing new products but also rethinking our entire approach to their design by asking questions we've been reluctant to ask about the materials we use—and being willing to change course when problems become apparent.

The news about the current state of the world is not good, but when it comes to the materials we use and the products we design, it is far from hopeless. Finding solutions depends considerably upon first understanding why such changes are necessary. Describing our future, Nobel Prize–winning chemist Paul Crutzen wrote in 2002, "A daunting task lies ahead for scientists and engineers to guide society towards environmentally sustainable management during the era of the Anthropocene," as he has dubbed our current geological era. "At this stage, however, we are still largely treading on *terra incognita*."[18]

That terrain has begun to be mapped. The chapters that follow explore some of that territory and investigate why its discovery is so urgent.

CHAPTER TWO

Swimmers, Hoppers, and Fliers

There is no sunrise or sunset. It is December 2007, nearly 350 miles north of the Arctic Circle. What light there is comes as a kind of twilight beginning as a deep cobalt blue shortly before noon and heightening to a liquid lilac before sinking back to darkness above a prism-edged horizon by 3:00 PM. Temperatures have been hovering all week around 0° F with wind chill down to almost –30 degrees. We are surrounded by ice in every direction as far as the eye can see. Our ship is the only one now at sea in the Arctic.

I took these notes while on board the CCGS *Amundsen*, the Canadian Coast Guard icebreaker and scientific research vessel on the first expedition ever to spend the winter moving through sea ice north of the Arctic Circle. The expedition had begun the previous July and was the largest of the 2007–2008 International Polar Year projects, involving more than 200 scientists from fifteen countries. Called the Circumpolar Flaw Lead System Study, the expedition's mission was to hug the lead of open water between the central sea ice pack—the ice that builds up and moves south from the Polar Ice Cap—and the coastal ice, a place particularly sensitive to environmental changes.

For almost a month, between late November and shortly before Christmas my home, shared with an international science crew of twenty and Coast Guard crew of forty-five, was a 300-foot-long floating laboratory capable of slicing through ice 1 meter thick. During those three-and-a-half weeks, we navigated the ice in the Amundsen Gulf, the westernmost reach of the Northwest Passage, some 90 miles south of the Polar Ice Cap. Conditions have been changing drastically here, and what happens in the far north, says expedition coleader Gary Stern, a senior scientist with Canada's Department of Fisheries and Oceans and professor at the University of Manitoba, may well be a harbinger of what's to come farther south.

One of the expedition's areas of scientific investigation is contaminants, and that's the primary reason I'm along. Even here, hundreds of miles from the nearest industrial or agricultural activity, the sea ice, ocean, and Arctic biota—the scientific term that takes in both flora and fauna—regularly yield evidence of elemental and synthetic chemical contamination. This contamination includes not only herbicides, fungicides, and pesticides—chemicals that are used in open air or that may have washed directly into rivers or released from factories as industrial effluent—but also metals, among them mercury (from both industrial and natural sources). It also includes flame retardants and water repellants, among other substances that are, at least in theory, incorporated into the materials of the products they're designed to enhance. Among the errant compounds now found regularly in the Arctic, for example, are brominated flame retardants, including those known as PBDEs (polybrominated diphenyl ethers) used widely in upholstery foam, textiles, and plastics.[1] Also routinely recorded in the far north—some at remarkably high levels—are perfluorinated compounds (PFCs) used as stain repellants, waterproofing agents, and industrial surfactants (think Scotchguard, Teflon, Gore-Tex, and the slick coating on paper used in food packaging such as pizza boxes, candy wrappers, and microwave popcorn bags).

These same compounds are now being detected in animals and people all over the world. A network of more than forty sampling sites on seven continents has found evidence of these environmentally persistent pollutants (synthetic chemicals that tend not to biodegrade or break down into nontoxic components)—a mix of pesticides, fossil fuel emissions, and industrial compounds—virtually everywhere it looked, from Antarctica, North America, Australia, and Africa to Iceland.[2] A recent five-year study conducted in U.S. national parks across the American West and Alaska found these same contaminants in the majority of its snow, soil, water, plant, and fish samples.[3] That pesticides or the contaminant associated with tailpipe and power-plant emissions are being found in the backcountry of Glacier, Olympic, and Denali national parks, while disconcerting, is not too difficult to understand. There are roads through and around the parks and, at least outside of Alaska, agriculture, weed, pest control, and commercial development are not that far away. But that the same sites, let alone the Arctic, would be contaminated with flame retardants or perfluorinated chemicals—associated primarily with products used indoors—or with PCBs and DDT, which have been out of use in the United States for about thirty years, is more perplexing.

"Anything released in the mid-latitudes travels rapidly north," Gary Stern, who leads the expedition science team dedicated to contaminants study, tells me one morning in his office aboard the *Amundsen*. Stern is chief scientist for Leg 4B, as this segment of the expedition is called, and he clearly relishes sharing his knowledge. Chief scientist is a position of serious responsibility on a research cruise—"cruise" being the scientific lingo for these voyages. The chief scientist coordinates the ship's route with the captain, decides when environmental sampling instruments can be deployed, and makes sure the expedition's science program stays on track and the science crew stays safe. On an international project like this one, there's the added challenge for everyone of working with different languages—we had five languages on this leg: English, French, Chinese, Spanish, and Catalan—and with scientists of varying experience. Stern's bespectacled gaze is generally intent and serious but he has a subtly impish grin. For the Coast Guard's dress-for-dinner Sundays, Gary wears a Northwest Territories sealskin vest that rather matches his walrus mustache. And he's happy to pose for photos wearing the enviable pair of huge, long-haired white Arctic wolf fur mittens and matching hat made for him by the mother of the Leg 4B wildlife monitor from the Inuvialuit village of Sachs Harbour. The admirable fur handwork and the two computers, one showing a map of current sea ice conditions, on Stern's shipboard desk form a tableau nicely indicative of early twenty-first-century Arctic culture. This is Stern's eighth trip to the Arctic since his first in 1997. An analytical chemist by training, Stern has worked on developing methods to analyze a persistent pesticide called toxaphene. Looking at the mechanisms of transport and trying to understand what happens to such pollutants as environmental conditions change, says Stern, "is what got me interested in the ecosystem aspects of climate change."

Talking to scientists on the *Amundsen*, I quickly learn that what makes understanding atmospheric and ocean circulation key to understanding the impacts of global warming is also essential to understanding the environmental fate of contaminants. Being in the Arctic, especially in winter when ice, light, and open water contrast so dramatically, it's easy to understand how important a role temperature plays in the physical, chemical, and biological fate of everything in the air and ocean. From our extreme northerly location it also became clear what a literally pivotal role the Arctic plays in determining global air and water quality.

Thanks to patterns of atmospheric and ocean circulation, pollutants washed into the sea or released into the air in the Northern Hemisphere—where the bulk of the world's population and industry are located—generally go north, moving from warmer to colder climates. Persistent pollutants also move through the Southern Hemisphere and are accumulating in Antarctic ice, but because there's less industry and human population there, there's been less intensive study in that part of the world. And it was the northern trajectory that brought this phenomenon to light.

It's not known when the first persistent synthetic chemical contaminants arrived in the Arctic, but this kind of pollution has been detected there on a regular basis since the 1960s. Beginning in the 1980s, studies have consistently found what are considered to be high levels of hazardous chemicals in both the Canadian and the European Arctic. "Everyone thought the Arctic was pristine, so we were taken aback to find such high contaminant levels in top predators," says Stern. These substances include pesticides, herbicides, and industrial compounds that are not used locally and that were clearly coming from someplace far away. There are some local sources of persistent pollutants in the Arctic—I visited one in Alaska, a site where U.S. military waste was abandoned—but, says Eric Dewailly, a professor of social and preventative medicine at Laval University who works with the International Network for Circumpolar Health Research, most synthetic chemicals of this type found here come "100 percent from the outside."[4]

To distinguish these substances from other pollutants cruising the world's air- and waterways—metals such as mercury or greenhouse gases, for example—these long-lasting synthetic chemicals are often referred to as "persistent organic pollutants," or POPs for short. Used in this way, "organic" means that the chemical compound contains one or more carbon atoms. Not all organic compounds are toxic or persistent. These characteristics are determined by the molecule's overall chemical composition and its structure. And not all of the synthetic chemicals that are escaping from consumer products and causing biological anomalies that can lead to health problems are persistent. For example, the constituents of some plastics now under intense scrutiny for their adverse health impacts—bisphenol A, which makes up polycarbonate plastics (clear refillable beverage and baby bottles, dishware, appliances, bike helmets, eyeglass lenses, food can liners, and dental sealants among countless other products) and the phthalates (pronounced "thalates") that make polyvinyl chloride (PVC) plastics flexible (shower curtains, toys, medical tubing, packaging, fabric coatings, to name but a very few)—are organic and potentially toxic, but do not last long enough in the environment to be considered persistent or to travel long distances.

Public awareness of POPs such as DDT, PCBs, and dioxins has been growing, but when not part of a calamitous tainted product incident, industrial accident, or alarming health discovery, they have rarely been the stuff of headline news. Yet by 2001 concern about the environmental and health impacts of POPs had risen sufficiently to prompt the United Nation's Environment Programme to have formulated a treaty called the

Stockholm Convention aimed at curtailing the use and release of these chemicals. "Exposure to Persistent Organic Pollutants (POPs) can lead serious health effects," writes the organization that administers the Stockholm Convention, "including certain cancers, birth defects, dysfunctional immune and reproductive systems, greater susceptibility to disease, and even diminished intelligence."[5] (The United States has signed, but as of May 2009 had not yet ratified, the Stockholm Convention—so it has not been a full participant in its meetings and decision making, and its use of chemicals is not yet formally bound by the Convention's regulations.)

Until now, the Stockholm Convention has covered only a dozen of the more than 80,000 chemicals that are sold commercially—PCBs, dioxins (which are a chemical byproduct rather than a substance formulated deliberately as a product ingredient), and ten pesticides. In May 2009, nine additional POPs were listed under the treaty.[6] Among these new substances are several brominated flame retardants and a perfluorinated compound and its breakdown products—substances known to enter the environment from finished products as well as industrial sites. Before these additions, none of the chemicals regulated by this international agreement were synthetics that emerge from consumer products. Still, what's currently regulated by the Stockholm Convention is but a fraction of the synthetic chemicals that persist in the environment, are bioaccumulative, and pose risks to human health.

These persistent synthetic chemical contaminants are now literally everywhere, and detecting, monitoring, and measuring their extent has become a worldwide scientific enterprise. This activity has grown to such a scale that more than a thousand participants from forty-six different countries gathered in Tokyo to share scientific information about these contaminants. On a steamy early September day, those of us attending Dioxin 2007 sat on closely arrayed chairs in a hotel ballroom where we were addressed by Japan's Imperial Highness the Crown Prince Naruhito. "Industry has given us a rich and convenient life," he told us. "But at the same time we're being faced with a new problem: degradation of the environment. Persistent and toxic chemicals that accumulate in the environment and persist on a global scale," he noted, are among our greatest problems. While this was not news to the conference audience, his Imperial Highness's statement seemed remarkable given that the highest levels of the U.S. government had spent much of the preceding decade resisting policies that would begin to deal with the magnitude of this issue.

Over the next three days I listened to a geographic smorgasbord of presentations. Researchers working on virtually every continent, in every ecosystem, shared findings about the presence and behavior of mobile synthetic chemicals with structures and compositions that create an array of environmental and health problems. The magnitude of what these scientists were finding was stunning; the audience was left with no doubt that these substances have permeated the world's environment and are interacting with our most fundamental biochemical mechanisms.

❖ ❖ ❖

It took three days, five plane flights, and one helicopter ride for me to get from my home in Portland, Oregon, to where the *Amundsen* was stationed in the Arctic Archipelago. Chemical molecules regularly travel farther without the aid of mechanical transport. I wanted to know how this was possible. I also wanted to know why the products of our rich and convenient life are turning up not only in U.S. national parks, but also in polar bears, deep sea squid, newborn babies, Japanese vegetables, eggs laid by hens in Belgian backyards, and packages of American cream cheese, along with most adults who've been tested, not to mention in more obvious sites of pollution like China's Pearl River Delta, the Great Lakes, and San Francisco Bay. I also wanted to get a glimpse of the part of the world on which they are having a significant impact and where environmental changes now underway will determine the effect of contaminants worldwide. So I headed north.

Inside, the ship is warm, dry, and brightly lit. The engines thrum constantly and work goes on twenty-four hours a day. With the loss of daylight, days seem suspended. Outside, beyond the double sets of heavy metal doors, the decks are covered with frost and fine crystalline snow. From my bunk-length berth on the lowest level of the ship, whenever we moved, the sound of breaking ice roared just beyond my porthole. An extraordinary grinding, creaking, and crashing sound, it was like being in the scoop of a giant snowplow.

Labs housing sophisticated analytical equipment are tucked into the corners of the ship, some accessible only from the chilly decks. A cold lab is kept at temperatures down to almost −15° F to preserve ice samples. Labs not much bigger than broom closets hold microscopes to view plankton and other tiny marine organisms, including viruses. There is indoor access to the Arctic Ocean through a kind of trap door in the base of the ship called the Moon Pool, where water sampling bottles and nets are lowered along with an elaborate instrument to measure turbulence. The ice beside the ship also becomes a laboratory. When ice conditions were stable, an "ice cage" could lower scientists and equipment by crane onto the ice about 25 feet below the *Amundsen*'s deck. Arctic research is clearly not for the weak. Heavy boxes holding ice corers—these resemble 4-foot-tall corkscrews that can extract poles of ice about 6 inches in diameter, samples that are an Arctic research staple—and other equipment are hauled out onto the ice. Work goes on in the short Arctic twilight and full dark, illuminated by the ship's powerful spotlights.

Clad in bright orange, insulated one-piece flotation suits, boots warm down to −40° F, big mittens and liner gloves, balaclavas, and hoods, the scientists maneuver their gear onto the ice and begin sampling. "What's the biggest challenge of Arctic winter fieldwork?" I ask. "The cold? The dark?" "Fingers," the scientists all say smiling. Big mittens keep hands warm, but many tasks require dexterity. To ensure I have the full experience, I am given small jobs: recording measurements, sealing sample bags, retrieving ice cores. I quickly agree without hesitation—fingers.

No one is allowed on the ice without a gun-bearer to keep watch for polar bears. Coast Guard crew are all qualified and several scientists have gun licenses but Trevor Lucas, our wildlife monitor for this leg of the expedition, is usually on duty equipped with rifle and two-way radio. A lifelong resident of the tiny Banks Island Inuvialuit community of Sachs Harbour, Trevor is in his thirties and has been hunting for about twenty years. One morning when we were on the ice in the gray blue dark, he turned to me and said, "Seals." Several hundred yards ahead in a spot of open water were several dark specks. Later from the bridge, I watched them through binoculars, as they popped their dark whiskered heads up for air and then dove back in.

The Canadian government issues a fact sheet detailing the contaminants regularly detected in ringed seals from this part of the Arctic. These seals, which are an important traditional food for residents of the Arctic, are known to contain pesticides, PCBs, and mercury along with PBDEs, PFCs, and other relatively new contaminants. On this dark season's leg of the expedition when wildlife is scarce and generally dormant, however, scientists focus on ice, water, and air samples, all of which will be tested for a suite of contaminants.

Ice cores are drilled, sawed into lengths, and put into coolers while we're on the ice. Some of the analysis will be done on the ship. Other samples will be sent to home labs where even more sophisticated equipment awaits. Each of these samples is a kind of snapshot in time, as researcher Jesse Carrie put it, and will provide data that help form one piece of the giant jigsaw puzzle from which a particular picture of the environment will emerge. Spending time with scientists doing this kind of field work, I came to think of their work as a pointillist painting in which each dot on the canvas represented a study that might be years in the planning and execution. It takes many such dots to create a panorama—a picture large enough to give a significant sense of what's happening over time, like the Intergovernmental Panel on Climate Change reports, for example.

The wintertime Arctic offers a vivid picture of the relationship between air and water that's key to both atmospheric circulation and the transport of contaminants. From where we were on the *Amundsen*, north of 70 degrees north, at the time of year when daylight wanes most dramatically and ice builds, it became abundantly clear how sensitive that environment is to changes in temperature, sunlight, and wind, and how open water can change everything. There were times when it was possible to see heat steaming out of the water—water that was −1° C into air that was about $-20°$ C. The stark contrast between the dusky white expanse of snow-covered ice and intense indigo water illustrated how ice acts like a blanket, regulating heat transfer between ocean and atmosphere. As expedition leader Dave Barber, who directs the Centre of Earth Observation Science at the University of Manitoba, puts it, "The ice is like a little 2-meter cap on top of 500 to 1500 meters of water. Take off the cap and the ocean is able to talk to the atmosphere."

What happens then can prompt a chain of cyclic events cascading across the hemisphere that can affect everything on the planet, from weather circling the globe to the tiniest organisms on Earth. Molecules of contaminants get swept up in this process as well. And some of these molecules, I'll learn later, borne aloft as aerosol particulates—very, very small solids—can influence cloud formation and precipitation, and thus contribute to the processes that set weather cycles in motion. Where a chemical ends up and how it travels depends on its molecular design and structure. This may sound obvious but these are behaviors that, historically, have been examined almost entirely after the fact—long after the horse has left the barn. Developing a systematic understanding of synthetic chemicals' mobility—a primary aim of green chemistry— can help us decide which materials we want populating our lives and landscapes.

By taking samples at numerous study sites over extended periods of time, scientists have discovered that some contaminants travel entirely by air—these are what Frank Wania of the University of Toronto calls fliers. Some—the swimmers—stay in the water, circulating with ocean currents. Most are hoppers, though; they make their way north in what's been dubbed the grasshopper effect, a series of air- and waterborne hops, moving toward the Arctic with cyclical and seasonal patterns of evaporation and condensation.

"Chemicals have several ways to be present in the atmosphere," explains Wania, speaking on the phone from his office. Depending on temperature and weather conditions, as well as the size, shape, and the elements that make up the molecule, the same substance can be found dissolved in water, as a gas, or as a particle. The smaller the molecule, the more volatile it typically is, and therefore the more likely to be swept along with atmospheric currents as a gas. These gas phase molecules—the fliers—can move in meters per second (spend time with scientists and even Americans end up speaking metric), making the trip from their points of origin to remote locations like the Arctic in days or weeks.[7] At the opposite extreme, the water-borne swimmers can take years to reach the same destination.

The hoppers, intermediate-sized molecules that can move between gas, liquid, and particle phase, may take days, weeks, or even years to reach the Arctic after their initial release somewhere in the Northern Hemisphere. These hoppers may be present in liquid water, but as temperatures warm they will evaporate to gas phase but then condense and return to join water when temperatures cool. They'll repeat this cycle over and over again, rising and falling—or hopping—with daily and seasonal patterns of warming and cooling. It's in this way that many persistent chemicals move with clouds and precipitation as storm systems and ocean currents circle the globe, and why temperature so strongly influence how and where pollutants travel.

Being able to estimate how fast a contaminant travels has made it possible for Wania and his colleagues to create models that predict contaminant behavior. These scenarios can be used to calculate where and when a mobile and persistent pollutant may end up and when to expect a contaminant's measurable decline once it's taken out of commercial use. Such measures also help scientists track the comparative health impacts of various chemicals both close to and far from their sources.

"Persistence and mobility is what makes something troublesome," says Wania. "It's a very difficult, laborious, and time-consuming process to prove toxicity, and by the time you have evidence it may be too late." If a substance is "persistent, highly mobile, and can't be contained, you have a problem you can't rectify," he tells me.

Another major influence on the movement and deposition of persistent pollutants is precipitation. Put simply, the more it rains or snows the more likely these contaminants are to wash out of clouds and be deposited on land, lakes, rivers, and oceans. In a recent paper Wania and colleague Torsten Meyer note, "Real substances affected by changes in rain rate include lindane, aldrin [both highly toxic and persistent pesticides], highly chlorinated PCBs, PBDEs, and some currently used pesticides."[8] When it's warmer, more of these substances will tend to evaporate again and join the cloud layer, and from there the cycle of condensation and precipitation begins again. When present as aerosol particulates, the contaminants may accelerate precipitation as water droplets coalesce around the tiny solids.

Increased precipitation caused by global warming will bring contaminants along with the moisture, notes Robie Macdonald, a research scientist with the Canadian Department of Fisheries and Oceans, and his colleagues. "Look at the effects of storms like [Hurricane] Katrina, where archived contaminants were released into a very important estuary," says Macdonald of the pollution that was washed into the Gulf of Mexico. "If there are more frequent and intense storms with climate change, poorly archived contaminants get released. This is what's been set in motion." Raining toxics sounds a bit extreme, but that's what it amounts to.

Whatever affects atmospheric and ocean circulation clearly plays an important role in where environmentally roving persistent pollutants end up. The big hemispheric wind and ocean patterns known as gyres and oscillations all play a part—as do more localized storm systems and currents. "These routes all seem to force contaminants released in Europe to the Arctic," explains Derek Muir, a senior scientist in aquatic ecosystems research with Environment Canada who specializes in contaminants. "Think about Chernobyl," Muir says by way of illustration. "The radioactivity there ended up in western Scandinavia where a lot of reindeer were sacrificed as a result. Other contaminants follow the same pathway north from Russia."[9]

What happens once pollutants reach the far north is very much influenced by where there is ice. Ice typically stabilizes contaminants and holds them in place until they're released again when temperatures rise high enough for melting to begin. Greenland, which Muir describes as "a big block of ice 3000 meters or more thick," appears to play a big role in fate of contaminants in the Arctic, Muir tells me. With the current accelerated melting of the Greenland Ice Sheet, it's likely that Greenland is now acting as a source of contaminants in the Arctic as well as a sink.

More evidence of glaciers releasing contaminants emerged recently with the discovery that Adélie penguins on the Western Antarctic Peninsula are being contaminated by a current source of DDT.[10] Since levels of DDT in the atmosphere have been declining, it would seem logical that amounts in exposed animals would also decline—especially in such a remote location. But levels in these penguins have remained the same, prompting a study that found glacial meltwater to be the source of the continued contamination.

Evidence of PCBs, pesticides, mercury, and other contaminants being released to the atmosphere with Arctic melting and erosion continues to emerge as well. On the east side of Greenland and across the Greenland Sea on the remote Norwegian islands of Svalbard that reach all the way up to 80 degrees north—in the path of air and water currents coming off of Greenland and the European mainland—levels of PCBs, PBDEs, and perfluorinated compounds have been found to be particularly high. Svalbard's polar bears have contaminant levels higher than bears on the west side of Greenland or in the Canadian Arctic, says Muir.

If global air and ocean currents generally tend to push pollutants released in North America toward the Arctic, when pollutants are released within range of the Atlantic Gulf Stream or get picked up by northerly air currents that also blow east, North American pollutants can be transported across the Atlantic toward Europe. Similarly, air masses may travel a northeasterly path from Asia across the Pacific to North America. The manufacture of chemicals, plastics, metals, cement, and electronics—and waste processing—all sources of persistent and hazardous pollutants, are clustered in southeastern China along with rapidly growing and urbanizing populations. This regional industrial effluent, combined with power-plant, tailpipe, and shipping emissions and dust resulting from construction and desertification, creates a potent maelstrom of contaminants. Thanks to the trans-Pacific air currents, pollutants released in China make tracks across the north Pacific toward the western United States and cause local air pollution health problems in Japan and Korea. Dust from China can reach California in as few as four days and makes a regular contribution to formation of Los Angeles smog.[11]

"There's definitely evidence that the Chinese mainland is a source of contaminants" that end up in North America, says Muir. NASA satellites are now able to track these transcontinental dust storms and those that are traveling to and from other continents—the phenomenon is world-wide—and concern over the health risks posed by the contaminants they carry has prompted the U.N. World Meteorological Organization to create a tracking and alert system to warn of serious airborne hazards.[12]

Where the globe-trotting chemicals originating in Asia come down to earth depends both on atmospheric conditions or weather and the molecules themselves. If sufficiently volatile, explains Muir, the persistent pollutants can move swiftly across the Pacific and on up to the Arctic. But the chemistry of some contaminants—those that are heavier and less volatile—causes them to drop out of the atmosphere into the northern Pacific Ocean where they may move slowly through the water or be taken up by fish and marine mammals. Persistent pollutants that include PCBs, brominated flame retardants, and perfluorinated compounds have been consistently found in fish, seals, whales, and fish eating birds along the Pacific coast over the past decade. "Fish can become their own transports of contaminants and fish-eating birds are known to excrete contaminants," says Robie Macdonald. "Migrating animals are not a huge transport mechanism but it's focused," he explains, "because they take the contaminants to where they feed and hatch their young."

Just as size and structure help determine how a chemical travels, molecular structure and composition also determine whether or not that substance will bind with soil, remobilize with groundwater or, when temperatures warm sufficiently, if it will be released again as a vapor. Molecular composition and structure also determine if a substance will be taken up by plants and animals, and if so how and to what effect. Understanding these pathways—and their environmental influences—is key to figuring out how a chemical will behave in the environment, how it will interact with the food web, and how people may be exposed.

The chemicals most likely to accumulate in plant and animal tissue and thus climb the food web are those that are fat-soluble. Lipophilic chemicals, as they're called scientifically, are working their way up the food web anywhere flora and fauna—including people—are exposed to such pollutants. Lipophilic literally means "fat loving," and this term is used to describe chemicals that have an affinity for and are soluble in fat. Materials with this property are also often persistent—that they are fat- rather than water-soluble makes them resist environmental degradation. And they are "bioaccumulative"—when they lodge in fat cells they can accumulate in plant or animal tissue as part of the fat reserves being stored for energy. When an animal burns fat for energy—this happens in people as well as in birds and fish—the fat cells release their contaminants, thus fat is both a source and sink of persistent pollutants.

There are multiple ways people may absorb a particular lipophilic chemical, however, which is one reason figuring out sources of human exposure to these contaminants is tricky. For example, people are exposed to brominated flame retardants through household dust but also through food they eat that has accumulated these chemicals in its fat. In the Arctic—where contaminants are aggregating and animals that are staples of the traditional Northern diet have large stores of fat—the potential for exposure is magnified. The region's top predators, polar bears and humans, have some of the world's highest exposures to these pollutants.

Conditions in the Arctic are now changing in ways that make the region more vulnerable to contaminants' effects and are increasing the potential for exposure elsewhere as well. Global warming is prompting changes that are increasing the load of contaminants in the Arctic and exacerbating their impacts—among them the effects of the Greenland Ice Sheet melt. When persistent chemicals reach the Arctic, they are typically held in place for long periods of time by permafrost and ice. As rising temperatures melt the ice and permafrost, the contaminants are released.

"Climate change has brought earlier spring and summer is lasting longer," Stern tells me one dark winter day. "There's also more precipitation and it's lasting longer." More rain and snow along with greater and faster snowmelt cause erosion along riverbanks, lakes, and coastlines. All of this is likely to wash soil-bound contaminant particulates into lakes, rivers, and the oceans along with whatever pollutants come with the pre-cipitation. This is already being seen in the Arctic Archipelago along the *Amundsen*'s route. "The permafrost has been melting really badly on Banks Island, especially near the inland lakes and along the coast," Trevor Lucas tells me.

"The system is complex," says Robie Macdonald, describing the pro-cesses at work in the arctic that contribute to the distribution of persistent pollutants. "A major concern," he explains, "is whether you have water as a liquid or water as a solid: ice." This sounds simple, but in the Arctic it makes, almost literally, a world of difference. In addition to the extent of Arctic ice and rate of melting, age of ice also matters. For the physical properties of sea ice change as it ages and these dynamics can affect the surrounding ecology profoundly.

The first few days I was on the *Amundsen* we moved swiftly through newly forming ice. When we moved through the same stretch of Beau-fort Sea several weeks later, we were nearly trapped by blocks of ice al-most 3 feet thick. To make headway we had to advance, retreat, and ad-vance again. This was all what's called first-year ice—ice that has formed during the immediate winter. What scientists are watching warily is the ratio between first-year and multiyear ice—ice that has lasted through at least one summer melt season and is, on average, thirteen years old. Multiyear ice is mostly water and dense like an ice cube from the fridge. New ice is laced with brine crystals—little pockets that can harbor life and possibly contaminants. The porous new ice melts faster than the old, fur-ther pushing the Arctic system from light to dark.

"Twenty years ago, multiyear ice made up about 60 percent of the Arctic Sea ice cover. There is only now half that much," Jinping Zhao of Ocean University in Quindao, China, explained to me on the *Amundsen*.[13] This sounds dramatic in the abstract, but it's even more impressive en-countered firsthand. Multiyear ice is arguably the old growth of ice. Mas-sive, hummocked, and imposing, it is—like an ancient forest—an ecosys-tem anchor. What's happening now as temperatures warm is roughly analogous to what happens when an ancient forest becomes riddled with clear-cuts.

❖ ❖ ❖

My time on the *Amundsen*, and in April 2008 on the USS *Knorr*—a Woods Hole Oceanographic Institution research vessel at sea for another International Polar Year expedition called ICEALOT, investigating air chemistry in the European Arctic—gave me a whole new respect for weather maps. What these charts revealed would determine both the ship's course—hence our safe passage—and each day's scientific activity.

On the *Knorr*, every morning began with a meeting at which the day's chart of storm systems—air currents, pressure systems, and temperature—were discussed. The cloud ceiling, the height of the planetary boundary layer, and the prevailing winds would all help the scientists decide how to deploy sampling instruments and figure out what streams of pollutants might be detected. Along with the data that make their way into civilian weather reports—plots of cold fronts and pressure ridges—ICEALOT scientists also had access to information from satellites that track anthropogenic pollutants. These data appeared schematically as variously colored plumes tracing carbon emissions, sulfur, and nitrogen compounds. It's with these pulses of greenhouse gases and smog-producing compounds that persistent pollutants also travel.

The chemical constituents of Arctic air masses influence both weather patterns and air quality, I learned from scientists on the ICEALOT expedition. It also had become evident that pollutants themselves, as they influence cloud formation and whether surfaces absorb or reflect light, are contributing to warming trends. Looking at the weather maps and listening to the scientists explain pollutants' behavior, I began to picture little footprint tracks of these chemicals streaming across open waters, the undulating coastlines, and mountain ranges, gathering in clouds, melting snow, and being absorbed by plants and animals along the way. But how were these substances getting into the atmosphere and oceans in the first place?

Industrial smokestacks, drainpipes, open air or water applications of substances designed to kill certain forms of life, along with leaks, spills, and waste emissions are, collectively, one dimension of the answer. But what about those traces of what amounts to bits of what my computer is made of, or my neighbors' carpet, or our car upholstery, and the material lining the insides of the local pizzeria's delivery boxes—how are they getting to the clouds and ocean?

Monica Danon-Schaffer is a chemical engineer at the University of British Columbia who is investigating how and why these kinds of chemicals are ending up in landfill leachate and water in the Canadian Arctic including north of the Arctic Circle. One of the great things about writing about science is its endless opportunities to inflict one's curiosity on people who are professionally curious. If you're lucky—as I have been—you find scientists who are as enthusiastic about explaining as you are eager to ask. Monica is one of those people.

We were in the Austin, Texas, airport waiting for early morning flights home after a conference. Though it's not even 7:00 AM and she's loaded down with backpack, hiking boots, and computer bag—luggage from an extended research trip up north—she whips a notebook out of her pack.

"Let me show you something," she says. In seconds Monica has sketched out of series of molecules—PCBs, PBDEs, a couple of perfluorinated compounds, and another kind of chemical called a short-chain chlorinated paraffin (used as industrial lubricants and coatings, among other applications). The PCBs and PBDEs are markedly similar: strongly bound carbon ring structures with either chlorine or bromine atoms attached. The chlorinated paraffin and PFCs also bear a striking resemblance: Both are made up of long, branching chains. Both of these shapes—the rings and these kinds of long interlocking chemical branches—are very sturdy and stable, Monica tells me. The very structure that makes these substances effective in squelching fire, effectively flexible, or adept at resisting moisture, for example, Monica explains, is what makes them so persistent. These molecules are strong and don't easily give up either their structure or its linked chemical activity. And as it turns out, this is also what them makes them incompatible with, or toxic to, some vital biological systems.

While these substances resist degradation persistently in the environment, because they are added to—mixed in—rather than chemically bound to the materials they're used to modify, eventually they become separated and leave the finished product. This is partly what makes it so difficult to keep track of and trace these chemicals environmentally. For one, exactly how much of each substance is produced is not precisely known. Nor is it known exactly how much goes into each product, let alone how much can be expected to separate out and when or where this happens. As I later learn, the mixtures of these chemicals used commercially are typically not 100-percent pure and so may contain other synthetics that finished products may also shed. Then there's the fact that, in the environment, many of these problematic synthetics break down into smaller molecules that may be more persistent or more toxic than their larger cousins.

Finally it dawns on me that what in one dimension is a design success—a new material that prevents upholstered furniture from bursting into flame or another that makes it possible to etch semiconductor circuits and prevent fabric from soaking up stains—may under other circumstances be a design flaw.

❖ ❖ ❖

An important thing to know about the scientific detective work of monitoring and measuring pollutants is that generally you will only find what you set out to look for. The methods for detecting particular chemicals in any form—gas, liquid or particulate—are very specific. While the same sample of ice, water, or air may yield an entire suite of contaminants, how one kind is detected may not be compatible with measuring another. As Tom Harner, a senior scientist with Environment Canada who specializes in hazardous air pollutants, explained to me, "Every persistent organic pollutant is different and unique. Every chemical is a different story. Because each chemical is unique, we can't investigate for a range of chemicals—we really have to do one at a time and look at each chemical's diversity of properties."

Atmospheric chemistry is painstaking work. Scientists spend most of the day staring at computer screens, logging in and analyzing data. It's quiet and not particularly visual or dramatic work. What it all means comes not in the collection of raw data but in later analysis, typically

using other sets of data to provide context and perspective. The more observations and data there are, the richer the picture of what's happening
environmentally. So we are here, cruising the Greenland, Norwegian, and
Barents Sea during spring ice melt—which this year allows the *Knorr* to go
farther north than she's ever been, just shy of the mid-April ice edge
above Svalbard, a couple of degrees beyond 80 degrees north. "No one
has been in this part of the Arctic at this time of year to take these kinds
of measurements before," Tim Bates and Patricia Quinn, chief scientists
for the ICEALOT cruise, tell me. The data gathered on board will help
the researchers understand if and how short-lived pollutants—particularly ozone, aerosols, and methane—are contributing to accelerated rates
of Arctic warming. These changes influence global weather patterns, and
hence the trajectory and impacts of these and other pollutants.

These contaminants reflect and absorb light and influence cloud formation and air chemistry in ways that can increase both atmospheric and
surface temperatures. Understanding how these pollutants behave and
contribute to warming in the Arctic—particularly in the spring, when sea
ice is decreasing and open water increasing—should help guide strategies
for reducing these impacts by curtailing the emissions that set these processes in motion.

While the scientists are logging data, I have plenty of time to explore
the ship. The library has a set of Patrick O'Brian novels, some thrillers,
and more highbrow fare ranging from John McPhee's books to Jared Dia-
mond's and Bruce Chatwin's. There are field guides to marine life, to
birds of the Southwest Pacific, the West Indies, and the Galapagos. There
are music dictionaries and books on geology. There is also a volume entitled *How to Abandon Ship*. "Do not hurry," it says. "A toothbrush will help
alleviate thirst, and carefully rationed whiskey or brandy is good for
morale."

The berth that Lynn Russell, a professor of atmospheric chemistry at
the Scripps Institution of Oceanography, and I have been assigned is below decks, across from the engine room. We sleep in shallow, narrow
metal bunks near a wall of heavy metal lockers and drawers. On top of
the lockers are orange life preservers, tubular sacks that contain survival

suits, and boxes that hold smoke hoods. At night the metal vibrates in a symphony that John Cage might have entitled *Work for Bandsaw, Electric Cello, and Cement Mixer*. For a couple of days we have heavy seas, with winds up at 35 knots and whitecaps that wash across the deck-level portholes. At one dinner, the usually boisterous and hungry science crew stares quietly and palely at bowls of spaghetti and meatballs.

After a couple of days along the north coast of Svalbard, where we can see the craggy, snow-covered fjords of Ny Alesund—where some of the longest-running, high-latitude records of persistent pollutants have been logged—we turn south toward Iceland along the east coast of Greenland. About 340 miles north of Iceland we pass Jan Mayen Island, the world's northernmost volcano, where by 1638 Dutch whalers had hunted the last of the local Greenland right whales to extinction. According to seafaring lore, an Irish monk named Brendan sailed close to the island in the sixth century, saw the fiery mountain surrounded by glaciers and freezing seas, and reported that he'd found the entrance to hell. When we sail by it's a snow-covered Mount Fuji rising from the sea against a clear blue sky. Gannets, gulls, skuas, and fulmars ride the turquoise-lit swells, likely carrying with them invisible loads of pollutants, some of which may be decades old.[14]

"We are seeing these chemicals in people and in biota where they shouldn't be," says Tom Harner. "With the newer generation of chemicals we're going at things a bit more quickly than we did with what we're now calling the 'legacy POPs,'" says Harner. "We're now trying to extrapolate from our existing knowledge base. Some models apply fairly well. For example, with PCBs and PBDEs, there's pretty good agreement on how these chemicals behave in the environment," he explains. I think of the molecules Monica Danon-Schaffer sketched out for me and how the PBDEs so strikingly resemble PCBs.

"But some of these compounds almost have two personalities," Harner continues. "In one phase they can be hydrophobic—resist water and prefer to partition or attach to fat—and so accumulate in fat tissue, soil, and plant cuticles. In other phases they can be hydrophilic—be water-soluble—and be transported that way." In other words, some compounds can hop, swim, and fly—behavior that is influenced both by the chemicals' structure and the physical landscape and atmospheric conditions that surround them.

Asking questions about how a chemical's structure will determine its behavior under various environmental conditions is a prerequisite of green chemistry. Had such questions been asked about PCBs or PBDEs— or had more attention been paid to the answers and their implications— they might not be turning up in birds cruising the northernmost fjords of Norway, for example. Similarly, had such questions been asked of some everyday plastics, their molecules might not be making less lengthy but no less significant journeys from products made from those materials to our bodies.

CHAPTER THREE

Laboratory Curiosities and Chemical Unknowns

It's before dawn on a chilly early spring morning and I'm sitting in front of a skyline mural in an otherwise empty rental TV studio in downtown Portland. I cannot see the news anchor who is somewhere on Eastern Standard Time but her voice in my ear says, "Coming up at the top of the hour, 'Do plastics make us fat?'"

I have just ninety seconds to unravel the hype and explain the research about endocrine-disrupting chemicals—as these synthetics are called because of their hormone-like effects—that I have recently written about for the *Washington Post*. Early in 2007, scientists gathered at the annual meeting of the American Association for the Advancement of Science (AAAS) announced that studies investigating the impacts of some widely used manufactured chemicals known to interfere with the body's system for regulating reproductive development, metabolism, and growth also appear to trigger fat-cell activity. That chemicals used in consumer products and at high volume all around the world might be linked to obesity—a health problem leading to numerous chronic diseases now at record levels in adults and children—had clearly caught news editors' attention.

The World Health Organization estimates that more than 1 billion adults worldwide are overweight and 300 million are obese. According to the U.S. Centers for Disease Control, about two-thirds of all American adults are now obese or overweight. Since the 1960s, the percentage of U.S. children aged six to eleven who are obese has doubled, and rates of obesity among adolescents have more than tripled, so that almost one in six Americans under age nineteen are now severely overweight.[1] Because obesity carries a risk of cardiovascular diseases, diabetes, stroke, and certain cancers among other adverse impacts, it is now a major health concern. Scientists have begun examining a wide range of possible causes beyond eating too much and exercising too little—including possible chemical exposures. The evidence is preliminary but all of the scientists I queried agreed that the findings on the potential contribution of endocrine disruptors to the rise in obesity had merit.

The synthetic chemicals under scrutiny that are apparently leaving finished products and making their way into our bodies are used to make products that range from marine paints and pesticides to plastic food and beverage containers—things we encounter every day. A spokesperson for the chemical industry dismissed the health-related concerns, but the scientific program administrator at the U.S. National Institute of Environmental Health Sciences (NIEHS), Jerry Heindel, who chaired the AAAS session, characterized the suspected link between obesity and exposure to endocrine disrupters as both "plausible and possible."

These obesity-linked studies were the latest additions to a steady stream of peer-reviewed articles published in scientific journals documenting the disturbing impacts of synthetic compounds that are leaching from consumer products into the environment, some traveling as far as the Arctic, finding their way via food, dust, air, and water into our bodies. Many questions remain unanswered, but well over a decade's worth of research suggests that these chemicals—which are also entering the environment from manufacturing and waste sites—are indeed capable of interfering with the hormones and cellular processes that regulate our metabolism, our sex organs, and our children's neurological and reproductive development. I'd been following this science pretty closely for several years but this new evidence was especially disconcerting.

What's become evident is that these manufactured materials have a structure and chemical composition that enable them to quite literally interfere with hormonal functions essential to keeping a human or other animal body healthy. The body's chemical messenger system, hormones work by sending chemical signals that prompt the processes responsible for nearly every bodily system. To do so, their molecular structure and chemistry has evolved to interact in very specific ways—and at very specific times—with receptors that trigger equally specific biochemical responses. The chemicals released in response set in motion much of what maintains a body's physiological homeostasis, its healthy balance.

With structures that are often strikingly similar to compounds that occur naturally within the body, synthetic chemicals characterized as endocrine disrupters can interfere with these processes by mimicking the behavior of naturally occurring hormones and thus blocking the body's own hormones from accessing the receptors that determine a host of vital bodily mechanisms. In this way, these manufactured compounds can disrupt how thyroid, estrogen, androgen, testosterone, and other hormones function. By causing their disruption, these alien substances— "xenobiotic" is the term scientists often use—can upset the finely balanced feedback loops that regulate metabolism, reproductive cycles, how a fetus develops, how a child grows, how a body's immune system responds to infection, and even how brain cells receive and send signals. "The endocrine system is very delicate and it doesn't take much to mess it up," explains the pioneering environmental health analyst Theo Colborn, who has researched endocrine-disrupting chemicals since the early 1990s.

Such chemicals now permeate the universe of twenty-first-century consumer products. They are used to grow, process, and package our food, and they are found in many appliances, electronics, and toys. They're in the materials used to construct our homes and cars, carpet our floors, and upholster our furniture. They are found in the synthetic fibers that make up most of our clothing, in numerous toiletries, cosmetics, and other personal care products, and in medicines to facilitate their delivery. These chemicals, says Linda Birnbaum, former director of the EPA's Division of Experimental Toxicology (and, as of January 2009, director of the National Institute of Environmental Health Sciences), "don't stay put in products," and thus give rise to a "global transboundary [pollution] problem." What kind of long-term harm are we potentially causing wildlife and ourselves by putting large quantities of these chemicals into our products? she asks.

The aesthetically fussy have long derided plastic as cheap and tacky.
The environmentally conscious consider it a symptom of our consumptive, landfill-clogging culture. But now more than style- and consumer-
consciousness are at stake: Use of these virtually inescapable synthetics
may be capable of harming the health of future generations. It's one
thing to insist on glass, china, or silverware at the dinner table. It's another to eschew plastics and synthetic fibers altogether. You may vow
never to use another plastic shopping bag or spoon again, but are you going to forgo your computer or cell phone? What about your bike helmet
or your child's car seat? Your contact lenses? Your toothbrush? No more
waterproof jackets?

Of course it's not just plastics; nor are all plastics or all synthetics per
se environmentally harmful and detrimental to human health any more
than are all chemicals. But how is it, I wondered, that we have built more
than several generations of products with synthetic materials whose
chemistry seems to be at such odds with ecological systems and with the
most fundamental workings of the human body?

✛ ✛ ✛

In 1955, a representative of the DuPont Company drafted a talk to the
Louisville Section of the National Association of Cost Accountants that
began, "I believe that most of you are familiar with our slogan 'Better
Things for Better Living—Through Chemistry.'" "Our Company depends
on its research program," he continued, "to provide new and improved
products—the 'Better Things' of our slogan. We have been proud to publicize the fact that more than 60 percent of our sales in 1950 resulted from
products which were unknown, or at least were only laboratory curiosities, as recently as 1930."[2]

In terms of technological innovation, 1930 seems light years ago. But
the chemical engineering work and materials choices of the 1930s—those
"unknowns" and "laboratory curiosities"—set our culture on the trajectory that has led, nearly eighty years later, to press conferences warning

consumers of health risks posed by vinyl shower curtains, to retailers discontinuing sales of shatterproof polycarbonate baby bottles, the analysis of waterproofing compounds in polar bears, and to the discovery of xenobiotically compromised immune systems in endangered sea turtles. For it was in the 1930s that chemical engineers at work in laboratories like those of DuPont's Pioneering Research Division were on what turned out to be successful quests for water-resistant wrapping materials, flexible films, and moldable, durable polymers.

Polymers are large molecules typically made up of many repeating smaller units that result in pliable structures. There are natural polymers but the ones under discussion are synthetic and exist nowhere in nature. These manufactured molecules have become ubiquitous in modern synthetics, in part because they lend themselves to creating surfaces resistant to heat, water, and other chemicals. Because polymers are physically large they have often been assumed to be unlikely to enter or interact biologically with living cells.

It was then—in the 1930s—that chemists designing products destined for mass-production began to shift their attention from synthetics based on cellulose, corn, milk, alcohol, and starch to materials built from petroleum products. The promise of these new hydrocarbon-based materials brought a decisive shift in the nascent industry of high-volume commercial synthetics—both in the United States and Europe—from bio-based materials to those constructed from petroleum and fossil fuel.

For anyone born after the 1950s, it's hard to imagine life without stretchy, clingy, transparent food wrapping, without plastic sandwich and freezer bags, and without store shelves filled with products packed in plastic jars, tubs, and tubes. We take waterproof, water-resistant, stain-repellant, stretchable, no-iron fabrics and lightweight, impressively durable plastics for granted. But in 1935, the design of a translucent, flexible, malleable, waterproof, and insect proof material had yet to be perfected.

Cellophane and some other polymers had already been invented. But without additives, cellophane—which is based on cellulose—and other films based on corn (zein), sugar, gelatin, and milk (casein) that DuPont and other companies (B. F. Goodrich, Goodyear, Phillips Petroleum, and

Standard Oil among them) were working with at the time are not inherently moisture-proof. Cellophane resists water, but is not impermeable to water vapor, which limits its applications considerably. DuPont had patented a moisture-proof cellophane in 1927, but nearly ten years later engineers were still working to design an improved cellophane-based polymer. They were trying to devise a material suitable for insect-proof biscuit wrapping that could be used as a sausage casing, and that was "tough" and "protective" enough under wet and cold conditions to be used for "packing iced goods, such as fish and other sea foods, or as a liner for wooden butter tubs" and milk bottle-cap liners.[3] Bigger-ticket items on the drawing board at the time included synthetics that could compete with and enhance natural rubber and that could serve—among other applications—as a material for electrical insulation and that could form pipes capable of carrying chemicals.

When reports of newly synthesized materials with an "absolute resistance to water and exceptionally high insulation properties" began to circulate in the mid-1930s among chemical engineers in the United States and Europe, they were discussed avidly. That these new compounds—among them chlorinated rubber and hydrocarbon products—apparently could be used in paints, as coatings for paper and metal, or could be spun into synthetic fibers and cloth, and could be readily shaped and molded, seemed especially attractive.[4]

Among these new compounds were "the first really practical high-grade synthetic materials which is [sic] a pure hydrocarbon," reported DuPont engineers. These synthetics, under development by a number of chemical and petroleum companies in the United States, England, and Germany, included one that became what we now know as polyvinyl chloride or PVC. (B. F. Goodrich is often credited with the development of commercially useful PVC, but as with subsequent generations of polymers, a number of competing similar products were developed more or less concurrently.) Now one of the most prevalent and versatile plastics, PVC accounts for nearly 90 percent of all plastics in use, according to one estimate, and is commonly used for commercial piping, to insulate electrical wiring, and was for years used as the basis for the cling-film food wrapping often generically referred to as Saran Wrap after the product first produced by the Dow Chemical Company. PVC has also been for decades the subject of controversy over its potential environmental and health impacts—adverse impacts that can occur during manufacture, use, and disposal.

The building block of this polymer had originally been discovered in the nineteenth century but it was brittle and rigid. The challenge was to devise a chemical design that would yield a product with the desired flexibility, strength, malleability, and moisture resistance. These qualities were ultimately achieved, beginning in the 1930s and 1940s, with the use of additives—plasticizing agents, solvents, and stabilizers. These ingredients often included the use of other petrochemical derivatives, along with chemical elements classified as halogens, primarily chlorine, fluorine, and bromine. In the case of PVC, these additives also included phthalates—a class of compounds now generally considered by scientists to be endocrine disrupters (a description chemical manufacturers dispute)—and sometimes lead, long known to be a neurotoxin. Thus manipulated, an incredibly useful base material was born, one that it's now hard to imagine the world without.

About twenty years later, toxicity concerns about PVC began to surface, but it wasn't until the 1960s and 1970s that the serious biological and health impacts of its chemical constituents—particularly the health impacts of the polyvinyl monomer from which PVC is built, now recognized as a human carcinogen—began to be discussed publicly, a discussion that continues today.[5] In the 1930s, the invention of this pliable, adaptable material known as PVC was a great leap forward. "These properties have allowed organic artificial masses to find application in a number of fields where hitherto natural products only were applicable," wrote DuPont engineers in 1936.[6] The invention of the hydrocarbon-based compounds that more or less began with PVC meant that such manufactured synthetics could now be fully substituted for naturally occurring materials. The material world would never be the same.

❖ ❖ ❖

It was no accident that many of the companies involved in chemical engineering in the 1930s were also in the petroleum business. The booming international petroleum industry provided a ready source of hydrocarbons. These byproducts of petroleum refining were consistent, plentiful, and as a feedstock or raw material for chemical products, inexpensive—all desirable attributes for ingredients of synthetics destined for mass production.

Throughout the 1930s, the price of oil remained stable at about $1 a barrel, and until the 1970s, petroleum prices did not rise much above $20 a barrel.[7] Apart from the escalation during the Arab oil embargo of the early 1970s and again in the early 1980s, the price of oil remained roughly between $20 to $40 per barrel until the precipitous price escalation that began in 2001 and ended abruptly with the 2008 financial market collapse and subsequent deepening recession. The generally low price and accessible high volumes of oil have played an enormous role in determining the synthetics that now populate our lives. Future price spikes and volatility seem inevitable, however, given finite oil supplies and their location.

The extent of our dependence on hydrocarbon-based materials, although barely a century old, is hard to fathom. There is virtually no aspect of twentieth century life that cannot now be linked to products that somehow rely on fossil fuels. "Up until about 1840, we were a wood-based culture," notes Christopher Reddy, a marine chemist at the Woods Hole Oceanographic Institute who has spent much of his career investigating the environmental impacts of oil spills and petroleum products. "After that there was an upswing in coal burning. Then right before 1920 there was a change to petroleum."[8]

In the spring of 2008, $4- to $5-a-gallon gas created a concatenation of the greatest acceleration of price increases in more than twenty-five years and affected everything from fresh produce to plastics. But until this spike in consumer prices, our petroleum dependence has largely been regarded as a given, not a choice to be reconsidered. "Oil provides the plastics and chemicals that are the bricks and mortar of contemporary civilization, a civilization that would collapse if the world's oil wells suddenly went dry," wrote Daniel Yergin in his epic history of the oil business, *The Prize*. For most of the twentieth century, Yergin observed in 1991, "growing reliance on petroleum was almost universally celebrated as a good, a symbol of human progress. But no longer. With the rise of the environmental movement, the basic tenets of industrial society are being challenged." This set the stage, says Yergin, for a great clash between "the powerful and increasing support for greater environmental protection" and the benefits of what he calls "Hydrocarbon Society."[9] Now, well into the first decade of the twenty-first century, between the impacts of petroleum-driven greenhouse gases and the biochemical impacts of petroleum-based synthetics, the full costs of "Hydrocarbon Society" are becoming painfully apparent.

❖ ❖ ❖

Public awareness of the far-reaching and long-lasting ecological and physiological impacts of environmental exposure to synthetic chemicals began, in many respects, to dawn with the publication of Rachel Carson's *Silent Spring* in 1962. But evidence that manufactured materials—materials designed to enhance and make human life easier—could also have impacts "totally outside the limits of biologic experience" had in fact been emerging since the mid-1940s, noted Carson.[10] "The chemicals to which life is asked to make its adjustment are no longer merely the calcium and silica and copper and all the rest of the minerals washed out of the rocks and carried in rivers to the sea; they are the synthetic creations of man's inventive mind, brewed in his laboratories, and having no counterparts in nature," she wrote. "Today we are concerned," Carson observed, with a "hazard we ourselves have introduced into our world as our modern way of life has evolved."[11]

By the 1960s, that exposure to certain widely used synthetics—particularly industrial chemicals and pesticides such as heptachlor, dieldrin, and aldrin—could result in acute and serious or even fatal illnesses had been known for years. Agricultural workers exposed to these chemicals suffered acute nervous system effects, some resulting in comas and blindness, while animals exposed tended to produce unviable offspring—litters and chicks that died soon after birth.[12] A number of these pesticides were suspected to be—and since have been classified as—possible or likely human carcinogens. That these substances have the ability to interfere with the chemical messengers or hormones that regulate metabolism and reproductive and physical development and help direct a body's immune and nervous systems began to be observed in studies during the 1950s and 1960s.[13] Throughout the 1960s, 1970s, and 1980s, as hundreds of newly synthesized compounds were launched into high-volume commercial production, evidence—from both lab experiments and field observations—continued to accumulate indicating that exposure to such chemicals could produce reproductive and developmental abnormalities.

Among the substances initially under scrutiny for their adverse biological impacts were insecticides (DDT among others), herbicides, industrial solvents, flame retardants, and manufacturing process chemicals such as PCBs. (In the case of pesticides and herbicides—materials designed to be lethal—the additional adverse impacts under study were to organisms other than targeted pests.) For the most part, these were compounds designed for industrial applications, and the first public or environmental health impacts of these compounds to be investigated were generally associated with open-air use—agricultural applications resulting in community exposure or food contamination, for example—or release of industrial waste.

What's changed substantially since the 1980s is the recognition that in addition to these well-known routes of contaminant release, individual consumer products—textiles, appliances, electronics, toys, packaging, personal care products, and so on—that contain synthetic chemical compounds can also be point sources of pollution. Indoor air along with household dust are likely to be the sources of a great many people's everyday exposure to such contaminants, Tom Harner of Environment Canada reminded me. This does not let industrial emitters off the hook but, as Harner says, offices and homes need to be considered emission sources for persistent and pervasive pollutants. Picture an aerial map of a metropolitan area and immediately you have a very different sense of point sources of pollution if homes and offices as well as industrial sites need to be considered.

In response to toxicity concerns raised beginning in the 1960s and 1970s, particularly about chemicals that can cause cancer, a number of once widely used synthetics have now generally—yet far from entirely—been taken out of use. Among these substances are PCBs, and a number of once widely used pesticides including DDT, dieldrin, lindane, mirex (also used as a fire retardant in plastics, paint, rubber, paper, and electronics), and toxaphene—all members of a class of chemical compounds called chlorinated hydrocarbons. Chlorinated hydrocarbons were, coincidentally, the synthetic compounds that proved so useful in formulating polyvinyl chloride and similar materials. And this is precisely the class of compounds that Rachel Carson singled out in *Silent Spring*.

About a dozen such synthetics (including the six named here) have been banned by the 2001 Stockholm Convention on Persistent Organic Pollutants, to which nine additional chemicals were added in May 2009. Yet the use of many synthetics long known to be toxic to human health and the environment—including those specifically restricted by the Stockholm Convention—continues, either unregulated (in the United States and many other countries) or through exemptions to existing regulations. Many of these substances remain in production, often in developing countries where workers and communities risk direct exposure. Furthermore, the past several decades' burgeoning global supply chains and streams of globally distributed products has created numerous additional potential pathways for these contaminants to travel.

Meanwhile, thanks to their environmental persistence, many chemicals released decades ago are still exposing us to harm. DDT and PCBs, dioxins, and other compounds restricted by the Stockholm Convention continue to contaminate. PCB contamination, for example, persists at many U.S. Superfund sites where cleanup is not complete and in places far from where they were originally used. PCBs are so persistent, explains Linda Birnbaum, that some 70 percent of all PCBs ever used are still somewhere in the environment.[14]

Current exposures to these older contaminants and to the subsequent generation of persistent pollutants—brominated flame retardants and perfluorinated compounds among them—are also occurring as these compounds are released from soil, water, snow, and ice. This is happening both where these chemicals were used or disposed of (often improperly) and where they have landed after years of environmental migration. The Alaskan village of Savoonga on St. Lawrence Island that I visited in July 2007, for example, is suffering from both types of persistent pollution: The village is a legacy site contaminated with PCBs and fuel oils and, at the same time, environmentally transported contaminants are entering residents' lives through the local wildlife food web. In addition, the effects of global warming now appear to be exacerbating the potential exposure and mobility of these persistent pollutants, both for banned compounds like PCBs and DDT and for succeeding generations of manufactured chemicals.

In the 1970s and 1980s evidence also began to accumulate that many of the synthetics under investigation or restricted because of potential carcinogenicity posed particular hazards to developmental and reproductive health. Since then these same compounds have been linked to additional health problems. There's increasing concern that learning problems, immune system problems, asthma, allergies, autoimmune diseases, and cardiac diseases may be influenced by exposure to these chemicals, particularly when that exposure occurs before birth.

"Today there is no such thing as no exposure," Birnbaum tells me. Yet simply because a chemical is present and measurable, she cautions, it's not necessarily a problem. "The problem is that we don't know. What you don't look for, you don't find," she says. "We may be looking too narrowly."[15]

Many synthetic compounds long in use and once deemed safe—polycarbonate and polyvinyl chloride plastics and the compounds that make now common waterproof, nonstick, and stain-resistant surfaces, to name just a few—are now being reexamined as potential environmental and health hazards. The net result is that since the 1960s and 1970s, despite ongoing efforts to regulate and restrict the use of synthetic chemical pollutants with potentially adverse biological impacts, we've added substantially to the mix of those that most of us are exposed to both daily and throughout our lives.

"The period between 1985 and 2000 to 2005 saw a ramping up of globalization, along with high-volume production of plastics, synthetics, and high tech products, which brought with it an explosion of new chemical products," says Derek Muir, a senior scientist with Environment Canada who specializes in the study of mobile pollutants. In the mid-1980s, the great boom in consumer electronics began, bringing with it a great surge in new chemicals, many designed or formulated specially to produce silicon wafers, semiconductors, and other components of high-tech electronics. The same period of time ushered in a huge international expansion in convenience and prepackaged foods along with supermarket and superstore merchandise ranging from personal care and cosmetics to easy-care fabrics and home-improvement products—much of which would not have been possible without synthetics. Between 1970 and 1985, one industry journal noted, some 65,000 new patents for polymers were registered, for an average of about 4,500 a year.[16] By 1990, between the collapse of the Soviet bloc and growing affluence in China, India, and other developing countries—thanks partly to the growth of high-tech manufacturing—synthetics-based, often short-lived consumer products were being produced and distributed at volume as never before. In 1962, Rachel Carson wrote in astonishment of the 500 new chemicals then being introduced each year. Today that figure would be about 2,000 new chemicals per year.

Of the 30,000 or more chemicals now used commercially in the United States and Canada, about 400 are currently recognized as persistent and bioaccumulative according to Muir and his colleagues. Only about 4 percent of these long-lasting commercial compounds with the ability to climb the food web are being studied on an ongoing basis, while about 75 percent of these potentially problematic compounds have not been studied at all, says Muir.[17]

There are entire categories of chemicals—polymers among them—now in widespread use that merit closer attention, in Muir's view. Typically, polymers are long molecules made up of a chain of similar, smaller units (picture a chain of interlocking identical and repeating links) that form plastics, resins, films, and surfacing and coating compounds—all materials on which our digital, portable, and disposable age has come to depend. As I'm taking notes over lunch with Muir during a conference break, I look around me in the shopping mall restaurant where we're sitting and take in the plastic tabletop, the disposable cutlery, the plastic drinking straw and lid on my iced tea, and little filmy packets of condiments. I notice the water-resistant book bag in which I've stashed my rainproof jacket, laptop computer, and cell phone. None of these synthetic products would be possible without polymers. Polycarbonate, PVC, and silicones (common ingredients in cookware, bendable plastics, and in personal care products like hair conditioner and lotions) are all polymers as are numerous other common plastics. Polymers are also made from the long-lasting perfluorinated compounds that go into materials that produce stain-resistant, nonstick, and waterproof surfaces used in consumer textiles and cookware as well as to make industrial films used in semiconductor production among other applications. But as Amy Cannon and other green chemists are showing with their development of nontoxic, fully biodegradable materials destined for products that range from high-tech electronics to food containers and cosmetics, a polymer need not be hazardous to be industrially and commercially useful.

Yet, Muir repeats, "Polymers have largely been ignored in terms of toxicity and this may be a problem for the future." This is another instance where asking the questions green chemistry advocates could prevent a problem before it occurs. Instead of creating polymers that break down into environmentally persistent, biologically active molecules with adverse health impacts, we should be able to design materials that will degrade innocuously and leave no toxic trail. While this new work gets underway, scientists all over the world are busy trying to understand the behavior of the problem materials with which we've filled the world.

CHAPTER FOUR

The Polycarbonate Problem

You can't taste it or smell it, but if you ate canned soup for lunch, drank a canned soda, or sipped from a refillable polycarbonate bottle—the hard, shiny plastic often labeled as #7—a chemical called bisphenol A may have entered your body.

More than 6 billion pounds of bisphenol A are now produced worldwide each year to make countless consumer products. As the chemical building block of polycarbonate plastics, bisphenol A is used to make hundreds of household items, among them food and beverage containers including baby bottles and toddlers' sippy cups, kitchen appliances such as coffee makers and food processors, sports gear, eyeglasses, CDs and DVDs, and electronic devices—including the exterior of the laptop computer I'm writing on now. Bisphenol A also forms epoxy resins, the thin plastic film used to line food and beverages cans—including those for soft drinks and infant formula—which are also applied as a dental sealant. It is a key ingredient of plastics with numerous other uses that include flooring, car parts, and water filters, and of a popular flame retardant used extensively in consumer electronics, textiles, paper, and many other products. In 2004, some 2.3 billion pounds of the compound were produced in the United States, most destined for plastics.[1] And before the September

2008 financial crash it was estimated that the worldwide annual consumption of bisphenol A would reach 12 billion pounds by 2011.[2]

The American Chemistry Council describes bisphenol A as "an industrial chemical used primarily to make polycarbonate plastic and epoxy resins—both of which are used in countless applications that make our lives easier, healthier, and safer, each and every day."[3] But rapidly accumulating scientific research indicates that bisphenol A is an endocrine disruptor and may be adversely affecting our ability to have children, our children's reproductive health, and even that of their children. Recent studies have also linked bisphenol A, which can mimic the hormone estrogen, to obesity, breast and prostate cancer, and to neurological problems.

Bisphenol A was first synthesized in the 1890s but the plastics made with it today were not developed until the 1940s and 1950s, and not launched into widespread commercial development until the 1960s. In the 1980s our use of these plastics really took off: Between 1980 and 2000, U.S. production of bisphenol A grew nearly five times. These ubiquitous plastics are big business. Sales of bisphenol A products, whose manufacturers include Bayer, Dow Chemical, and General Electric/SABIC, generate billions of dollars annually.[4]

Look around a typical early twenty-first century home—including the kitchen, bathroom, and children's rooms—and you'll find a lot of polycarbonate plastics. (A number of manufacturers make different polycarbonate formulations for varying applications, but all polycarbonates are bisphenol A–based polymers.) For decades, bisphenol A (BPA) has been used in what are called "food contact" consumer products as approved by the U.S. Food and Drug Administration and comparable agencies in Europe and Japan. Until recently, these government agencies were unequivocal in their safety assurances for polycarbonate plastic products. They have maintained, as does the trade association of manufacturers that produce BPA, that these products "are safe for their intended uses and pose no known risks to human health."[5] But a growing number of scientists disagree with this assessment, and news of their findings have thrust the compound into the center of a controversy that is challenging both the wisdom of unrestricted use of BPA and long established methods of determining chemical safety.

"Exposure to bisphenol A is continuous," says Frederick vom Saal, a professor of biological sciences at the University of Missouri at Columbia who has studied suspected endocrine disrupters, including bisphenol A, for about two decades. Vom Saal's work—particularly his discovery of the low levels at which bisphenol A appears to be biologically active—has made him one of the leading researchers in this field. His research has also drawn criticism from the chemical industry precisely because it upends assumptions on which the claims of BPA safety have rested.

Vom Saal explains that the source of BPA's recent notoriety lies in an apparent paradox: While the plastics in which bisphenol A has been a critical ingredient are strong, the chemical bonds that hold bisphenol A molecules together within these polymers tend to be unstable. Consequently, as the plastics age or become worn, bits of the polymer material—in this case bisphenol A—become detached. This makes polycarbonate capable of "continuous [BPA] leaching," says vom Saal. Since these plastics are now virtually everywhere, he continues, our exposure to the biologically active forms of their chemical components is also virtually ongoing.

Bisphenol A is used so widely that even if we're not eating food that's come into contact with these plastics, the substance is likely to be in our indoor air—the result of leaching from appliances, electronics, and other polycarbonate surfaces.[6] Errant bits of bisphenol A have also been detected in streams, rivers, and bays where wastewater is discharged and have been found leaching from landfills. A 2008 paper in the journal *Reproductive Toxicology* notes that as a result of such contaminant pathways—and the fact that BPA is not eliminated by current wastewater treatment methods—bisphenol A is likely also to be in water used for drinking and bathing.[7]

A U.S. Centers for Disease Control nationwide contaminants monitoring program has found bisphenol A in the blood and urine of 95 percent of the Americans tested, at levels *at* or above those that affect development in animals.[8] In research released in 2007, comparable levels of bisphenol A were found leaching from epoxy-lined food cans—including canned infant formula—tested by the Environmental Working Group, a Washington, D.C.–based nonprofit advocacy group.[9] Similar testing of food cans done in the early 1990s also yielded levels of bisphenol A high enough to produce cellular abnormalities.[10] Studies published in 2003 and 2006 found bisphenol A in the majority of indoor air samples tested, including virtually all air samples taken from daycare centers.[11] A Health Canada study released in early 2009 found BPA in 96 percent of the canned soft drinks tested—a study that covered 84 percent of all soft drinks sold in Canada—at levels below current government safety standards but that are, in hormone-exposure terms, equivalent to 500 times what are considered normal estrogen levels.[12] And a study led by researchers at the Harvard School of Public Health, published in May 2009, found that one week of polycarbonate bottle use increased urinary concentrations of bisphenol A by two-thirds.[13]

"Everyone is exposed to it. There's no doubt about that," says Dr. Hugh S. Taylor a reproductive endocrinologist at Yale University School of Medicine who is studying the impact of bisphenol A on female reproductive health.[14]

❖ ❖ ❖

Although it's only in the past few years that news of bisphenol A's health impacts began to reach a nonscientific general public—news that has since spread rapidly—it was first recognized as a synthetic estrogen in the 1930s. Papers published in the journal *Nature* in 1933 and 1936 describe its estrogenic effects on lab rats. These papers also commented on the possible carcinogenic activity of materials with similar or comparable chemical composition and structure to bisphenol A—specifically materials synthesized from petroleum (from which bisphenol A is ultimately derived) and coal tar.[15]

Some two decades later, bisphenol A was launched into everyday life with the development of commercially produced polycarbonates. Major production of these plastics began in the United States in the late 1950s after a General Electric engineer named Daniel W. Fox formulated a material based on BPA that GE called Lexan. The invention was not so much deliberately planned as it was the result of what Fox called his ability to take "a few clues and jump to conclusions that frequently panned out."[16]

While experimenting with different materials that might ultimately make a good moldable polymer, Fox decided to work with bisphenols, compounds derived from petroleum processing that were then being used to make various epoxy resins. As molecules, bisphenols have a structural feature that makes them useful as potential chemical building blocks. Attached to their hydrocarbon ring is what's called a hydroxyl group, an oxygen and hydrogen that together form a site to which other molecules can bond. This structure is common to both synthetic and naturally occurring compounds, a coincidence that will later turn out to be important to how bisphenol A behaves.

Fox's interest in the hydroxyl group was as a polymer building site, not for its biological activity. But when attached to a hydrocarbon ring as it is in bisphenol A, the entire chemical grouping becomes a molecule known as a phenol—an aromatic hydrocarbon, a ring made up of six carbon atoms and five hydrogen atoms plus a hydroxyl group. Phenols are commonly made by oxidizing benzene, which essentially means adding oxygen to benzene. Phenols are toxic, but they are also known for their antiseptic properties and so were used to kill germs in some nineteenth-century surgical procedures.

This molecular group consisting of six carbon-five hydrogen rings with a hydroxyl group attached, however, is also part of the structure of substances produced naturally by the human body, compounds that include estrogen and thyroid hormones. Introducing a manufactured chemical that includes the phenol group into a cellular environment may therefore pose a problem because the synthetic material may compete biochemically with the similarly structured naturally occurring chemical. Thinking in green chemistry terms, the presence of a phenol group on a synthetic, therefore, should be a sign to investigate that substance's potential as an endocrine disruptor.

The potential cellular toxicity of phenols has actually been known for decades. Research done in the 1950s, written about by Rachel Carson in *Silent Spring*, discussed the mechanisms by which pesticides constructed with phenols had the ability to prompt oxidation processes that upset cellular metabolism. These reactive chemical groups can disrupt formation of enzymes vital to energy production, which in turn may interfere with how an organism produces and differentiates cellular material. These processes of cellular reproduction are involved in virtually every bodily system, from how an individual processes sugars and calcium to how its reproductive system functions. Carson described the introduction of xeniobiotic phenols as thrusting "a crowbar into the spokes of a wheel."[17] Had Fox been a green chemist, our current synthetic landscape might look very different.

But because Fox and his colleagues were focused on functional performance and on working with readily available chemical ingredients, bisphenols seemed a good choice. As an additional building block that might combine with the bisphenol molecules' hydrocarbons to yield a useful polymer, Fox chose a chlorine compound called carbonyl chloride. Carbonyl chloride was then—and is currently—a common ingredient in the synthetics known as isocyanates that are used to make any number of products, including polyurethanes that go into varnishes, paints, and plastic foams. By the 1950s, it was known that chlorinated hydrocarbons made useful synthetics so this was a logical route for Fox to follow—but no one had yet made the kind of moldable, shatter-resistant plastic that Lexan turned out to be.

If you're building a polymer, a linked chemical chain in effect, you need lots of the same repeating pieces; ideally you'll work with shapes that are easy to find and lend themselves to chemical bonding. It's here that a Tinkertoy or Lego analogy comes to mind. To add pieces to a chemical structure, you need sites where new sticks and building blocks can be attached. So it was with the choice of bisphenols and carbonyl chloride, which lend themselves to such bonding and were both readily available industrial chemicals. Had Fox been practicing green chemistry, however, he would never—even with what was known in the 1950s— have launched a product that required copious quantities of carbonyl chloride.

Carbonyl chloride is also known as phosgene and is so toxic that it was used as a chemical weapon during World War I. The isocyanates it's used to make are also highly toxic. One such compound, methyl isocyanate, was the gas involved in the deadly 1984 disaster at the Union Carbide plant in Bhopal, India. Lest anyone wonder if nerve gas is lurking in your bike helmet or CD cases, however, let me quickly explain that no phosgene or even any chlorine ends up in the final bisphenol A polymer; the chlorine compound is simply a reagent, an ingredient that enables the desired chemical bonding to take place.

Yet speaking to an interviewer in 1983, Fox acknowledged that using large quantities of a chemical such a phosgene was indeed hazardous. But, Fox continued, it "was not a totally frightening undertaking because we had good advice. I would say that we have been tightening up our whole phosgene handling ever since, investing an awful lot of money in trying to make the stuff doubly safe and then triply safe and quadruply safe." Still, the interviewer pressed, "Has there ever been a problem?" To which Fox responded, "We have had one or two small discharges. To my knowledge, I don't think GE has advertised it, but I think we probably had a 'casualty' from phosgene." Did this give anyone second thoughts about going into the business? "I don't really think it did," Fox replied.[18]

At the time Fox was working, new material inventions like polycarbonates were just that—inventions that came first, with applications and markets found later. "When we invented polycarbonates in the early 1950s we had a polymer with an interesting set of properties and no readily apparent applications," Fox said in 1983.[19] But what was known about polycarbonates' behavior early on that might have hinted at what's since been discovered about their physical and biological behavior? Could this information have been used to prevent what are clearly problems of chemical contamination? Endocrine-disruption science is relatively new, but some of what was known early on about bisphenol A and polycarbonates would seem to indicate a material perhaps not ideally suited for use, say, with food, heat, and dishwashing detergents.

That polycarbonates built from bisphenol A were vulnerable to certain detergents, solvents, and alkali solutions (household ammonia would qualify) has been known since at least the 1970s. Ammonium hydroxide (essentially a solution of ammonia in water) was discussed as a possible way to break polycarbonates down into its chemical constituents—for materials recovery and reuse and as a way to remove unwanted polycarbonate from another surface. It was also known that various additives used to modify polycarbonate mixtures could leach from the finished plastics when they came in contact with certain liquids. Documents filed with the Federal Register in 1977 list chloroform, methylene chloride, and chlorobenzene among these additives.[20] (The U.S. Department of Health and Human Services considers chloroform and methylene chloride suspected carcinogens, while chlorobenzene is known to cause liver, kidney, and nervous system damage and produce a precancerous condition in lab rats.[21]) Correspondence between GE Plastics Division personnel in the 1970s and 1980s also voiced concern over the presence of chlorobenzene in water stored in polycarbonate bottles (but not bottles made by GE as it happened) and about how the stability of these polymers might affect their ability to be used with food.

A memo circulated within the Lexan division of GE in 1978 also noted that "through reaction with water," polycarbonate resin can degrade. "The two largest applications of Lexan resin for which hydrolytic stability is critically important are baby bottles and milk and water bottles," ran the 1978 memo.

In each application the finished parts are subjected to conditions which will cause, after prolonged treatment, molecular weight reduction. However, in each application, actual product failure is usually observed before significant molecular weight reduction is detectable by the usual techniques. . . . Baby bottles are subjected to autoclaving at 250°F in saturated steam and fail under these conditions by becoming opaque, and sometimes by shrinking and deforming. Milk and water bottles are washed in aqueous solutions of alkaline or caustic cleaning agents and fail by stress cracking. The relationship between practical failure modes and the fundamental physical and chemical processes involved is not fully understood.[22]

That polycarbonates might degrade when heated, washed, or exposed to sunlight was also discussed in company memos in the late 1970s and early 1980s. Three decades later, the plastics industry assures consumers that such wear and tear of polycarbonate baby bottles poses no health concerns for infant users.[23]

While developing a bisphenol A-based polycarbonate destined for frozen-food packaging with the freezer-to-oven market in mind, GE tested the new material's durability—including its potential to leach bisphenol A—under various conditions, including different oven temperatures. "BPA migration less than 50 ppb [parts per billion]" ran a 1983 memo noting the results. (The best visual capture of "parts per billion" I've heard is that one part per billion is the equivalent of one pancake in a stack of a billion.) The EPA's safety standard for daily bisphenol A exposure was set at 50 parts per billion in the late 1980s, despite the fact that testing done by and for the National Toxicology Program had already shown elevated instances of reproductive problems as well as higher-than-normal incidence of certain cancers along with liver and kidney disease in lab animals exposed to bisphenol A.[24] This safety standard continues to be used, despite subsequent research and the fact that the initial study—conducted in the 1970s—was done under what the General Accounting Office—the U.S. federal government's "watchdog" agency—considered to be poor laboratory conditions.[25]

That bisphenol A could leach from polycarbonate—and that it might not be entirely biologically inert—has thus been known for at least two decades. But it was not identified explicitly as an endocrine disrupter until the early 1990s. Like the initial invention of this highly useful and marketable polymer, one of the first discoveries of its endocrine effects was serendipitous. In 1993, researchers at Stanford University Medical School published a paper documenting the unexpected estrogenic effects they'd observed in an experiment—effects they eventually traced not to an intentionally introduced hormone or other substance but to a contaminant, which had apparently leached from lab equipment. That contaminant was identified as bisphenol A.[26]

That remarkably low levels of exposure to BPA could cause hormonal abnormalities and do so at the genetic level—thus setting the stage for multigenerational adverse impacts—was discovered by a similar accident. In 1998, Patricia Hunt, now professor of molecular biosciences at Washington State University, and her colleagues at Case Western Reserve University were investigating chromosomal changes that occur in egg cells. "We were trying to understand how age affects human eggs," Hunt told me.[27] The experiment, she explained, was designed to compare mice with abnormalities to normal—or control—mice. "One day the controls went bananas, showing a huge number of chromosomal abnormalities," recalls Hunt. The spike was so severe the researchers thought it must be caused by a sudden chemical exposure, "something in the air." Eventually, they figured out that the contamination was bisphenol A, released by degrading plastic in the mouse cages. Hunt and her colleagues discovered that a different kind of detergent than usual had been used on the cages, one that eventually caused the polycarbonate to become sticky. "Every cage and every water bottle had to be replaced and it took about a year to clean up," says Hunt. What she and her colleagues learned from the mess was that very low levels of bisphenol A were apparently responsible for causing serious abnormalities in mouse egg cells.

Hundreds of bisphenol A studies undertaken since these accidental discoveries have shown that the apparent endocrine-disrupting effects of bisphenol A include not only interference with egg cell and reproductive development, but also with neurological processes, thyroid hormone function, and metabolism—how a body processes insulin and maintains fat cells. There is also evidence that exposure to bisphenol A can alter immune system function, as well as suspicion that under certain conditions bisphenol A's biochemical effects can set the stage for the promotion of prostate and breast cancer.[28] What is of particular concern, in terms of health impacts, is that the most profound effects of bisphenol A appear to take place prenatally and in the early stages of development after birth—timing that can have a lifelong impact on an individual's health.

Particularly remarkable about these findings—and upsetting to traditional toxicology, which correlates level of adverse impact to size of dose or length of exposure, is that bisphenol A can produce these effect at what Frederick vom Saal calls "phenomenally small amounts."[29] Historically, material safety assessments have been based on the assumption that the larger the dose, the greater the effect. But because bisphenol A interacts with the endocrine system—a delicate and finely tuned series of biochemically triggered feedback loops—it responds to chemical interference in ways that confound traditional tenets of toxicology. As Andrea Gore, professor of pharmacology and toxicology at the University of Texas at Austin notes, "endocrine effects can happen at very low doses whereas high doses can have no effect at all."[30]

How new materials—including many of the synthetics that now populate our lives—have typically been assessed for safety during product development is illustrated clearly by the story of a bisphenol A–based polycarbonate called Daxus that GE devised in the 1980s. By building a polymer in a different way than the standard BPA-based Lexan polycarbonate and combining it with another polymer known as a polysulfone, GE created a material with the potential to withstand high levels of heat. This gave it promise for what GE company memos called "disposable cookware applications," the target being the suddenly booming early 1980s market in upscale frozen dinners—precooked meals packaged on little white plastic dishes that could go from freezer to microwave or conventional oven.[31]

Performance was paramount. The dishes could not melt before dinner was cooked. There are numerous internal memos documenting the precise temperatures and cooking times the polymer could withstand before dish edges began to curl and buckle. The safety protocols employed at the time to test for biological impacts seem, in retrospect, far less tailored to the product's specific applications—namely home oven and the dinner table—than do the performance tests, however. High-dose animal toxicity tests were performed. The scientific and industrial literature was searched for any record of the compound's adverse behavior. The latter yielded virtually no results (not surprisingly because it had just been invented), and earlier in-house testing detected no leaching of potentially hazardous substances, so it was assumed that the newly synthesized material had a clean bill of health. Some twenty years later, however, researchers at the University of Missouri determined that bisphenol A was indeed leaching from animal cages made from polysulfone—a key ingredient of this cookware.[32]

What no one was looking for in the early 1980s, when the first generation of microwavers were heating prefab dinners—and what standard toxicology still does not accommodate—was the possibility that low doses of an endocrine-disrupting compound like bisphenol A might produce an adverse (or toxic) effect even though a high does may not. Further confounding ideas of traditional toxicology is that time of such exposure—rather than length of exposure—to bisphenol A and other endocrine disrupters appears critical to the consequences of the impact. (Traditional toxicology looks at how long rather than *when* in an individual's life exposure occurs.) What makes this so significant is that as Hunt, Taylor, vom Saal, Theo Colborn, and other scientists studying endocrine disruptors explained to me, low levels of exposure during fetal development can cause lasting changes in reproductive and metabolic—even neural—development. These changes to the fetus are permanent and irreversible. (Impacts of adult exposure to bisphenol A, however, seem to be reversible, at least as tested so far.) "The fetus is exquisitely sensitive to bisphenol A. One hit during a brief window of time can influence future development," says Hunt.

In January 2007, Hunt and colleagues published a study showing that exposure to "environmentally relevant"—or available—levels of bisphenol A (what people might encounter through products used routinely) can disrupt normal egg cell growth in a developing female mouse embryo. Bisphenol A appears to affect very specific genetic receptors that prompt chromosomal abnormalities in the egg cells—affecting their mechanism for division and replication in ways that make them unviable—setting the stage for potential miscarriage.[33] Bisphenol A can thus affect three generations at once—the mother, who takes in the chemical; then her developing fetus through her; and if that is a female, then that daughter's potential children (via the egg cells) developing within that fetus.

Hugh Taylor and his colleagues have also seen lifelong changes in animals caused by prenatal exposure to bisphenol A. In a 2007 paper they show that exposure to bisphenol A during pregnancy can cause "lasting changes in development of the uterus that could pose problems during pregnancy," including potential miscarriage.[34] Is it possible, I asked Hunt and Taylor, that bisphenol A could be having comparable effects on people?

Both quickly explained that many factors contribute to miscarriage and other fertility problems.[35] "We're now seeing increasing fertility problems and it seems as if environmental agents could be a contributing factor," said Taylor who in addition to conducting research is an attending physician in the Department of Obstetrics and Gynecology at Yale–New Haven Hospital. "A lot of evidence points in that direction," he said. A difficulty in pinpointing cause and effect with these kinds of reproductive problems, Taylor continued, is that people don't know they've been exposed and the effects of exposure may not manifest themselves until twenty to thirty years later. "Environmental estrogens can alter the development of the reproductive tract in ways that can be subtle and hard to detect," he explained.[36] Comments Hunt: "To me any chemical that can mimic the activity of estrogen is scary."[37]

To date, all the in vivo endocrine system studies of bisphenol A have been animal studies. But Hunt, Taylor, vom Saal, and other scientists conducting endocrine-system research all explain to me that the genetic mechanisms affected by bisphenol A—including the basic processes of egg development—work virtually the same way in all animals, including people. This has led a panel of experts in endocrine-hormone research—a group of more than two dozen scientists that includes senior researchers with the EPA and the National Institute of Environmental Health Sciences—to say with confidence that the similarity of effects observed in wildlife and laboratory animals exposed to bisphenol A would predict that similar effects are also occurring in humans.[38] "We know enough to know that we should be concerned," says Hunt. "If we wait for comparable human data and it comes out like animal data," she adds, "we aren't going to be breeding as a species."[39]

❖ ❖ ❖

Looking back at the very early history of bisphenol A, that the compound would affect reproductive development would come to light as it did only in the 1990s seems surprising. For in the 1930s—about the time that the substance's estrogenic activity was written about in the journal *Nature*—bisphenol A was considered for possible pharmaceutical use as a synthetic estrogen but put aside in favor of a more powerful synthetic based on coal tar (rather than petroleum) products—a compound called diethylstilbestrol or DES. DES was developed as a pharmaceutical and prescribed to prevent miscarriage or premature deliveries from 1938 until

1971, when it was withdrawn after being linked to an unusual form of cervical and vaginal cancer, particularly in young women. Taken by between 5 and 10 million women in the United States, DES was also approved by the U.S. Food and Drug Administration as a growth hormone for livestock and was used to fatten cattle and sheep from the mid-1950s until the 1970s.[40] After its link to human cancers became known, concerns were raised about the ultimate effect on humans of DES use in cattle and the synthetic was banned for used with livestock in 1979, at which time other synthetic estrogens took its place in the meat industry.[41]

What was particularly striking about the unintentional effects of DES, explains Retha Newbold, a developmental biologist at the U.S. National Institute of Environmental Health Sciences who has spent over thirty years studying DES, is that it caused reproductive abnormalities in the children and grandchildren of women who took it—similar to the effects of bisphenol A exposure in mice observed by Pat Hunt and colleagues.[42] Investigating these impacts further, researchers discovered that the effects of endocrine disruption could be imprinted upon genes during development. This discovery is what scientists describe as an epigenetic effect, the alteration of a gene—often by introduction of chemical foreign to the body—that changes the way that gene will interact with other molecules in the cell's nucleus. This in turn will determine the biochemical signals that prompt how other genes are sequenced and how specific proteins are produced, all of which has profound effects on how an individual develops.[43]

Medical dictionaries define epigenetics as changes in gene function that occur without changing the sequence of DNA. This is an important distinction to bear in mind when considering the impacts of environmental chemical exposure. What this means is that it's possible, by changing the biochemical environment of a cell, to alter how a gene functions throughout that individual's life—perhaps also influencing that individual's children's hormone feedback loops—all without genetic mutation. Exposure that occurs early in life—particularly before or just after birth—seems to be a prime time for causing such changes, changes that set the stage for ongoing health problems, not only in infancy and childhood but also later in life. These changes may not cause problems for every individual: As Linda Birnbaum points out, we don't know if they will or not but it's important to know that these effects can occur. It's also important to remember that we are all exposed, not just to one chemical at a time that may prompt such impacts but to mixtures of these chemicals, both in time and in space, which may have additional adverse effects.

What this means in terms of toxicology is that just because a substance is ruled out as a mutagen—likelihood of mutation being a criteria routinely included in chemical safety testing—it does not guarantee that the substance it will not alter genetic function. Testing for epigenetic effects, however, is not currently part of official toxicological screening assessments. "New science," comments John Peterson Myers, "is overturning old assumptions about genes and the environment."[44] When genetically programmed health defects or impacts occur, he explains, it's not because you inherited "the wrong gene. That gene likely has been altered." When it comes to screening manufactured chemicals for such effects or protecting people from their consequences, "Today's health standards are too weak," Myers believes. "They're in the scientific Jurassic," he quips. But "if we modernize health standards, we can prevent diseases caused by non persistent chemicals" (such as bisphenol A).

❖ ❖ ❖

In the summer of 2007 a group of environmental health experts and internationally recognized scientists who specialize in endocrine disruption research, along with specialists in developmental biology, pediatrics, and toxicology, met in the Faroe Islands to discuss the perturbing findings of their work and to formulate a call for increased efforts to prevent prenatal and childhood exposure to chemical contaminants—efforts that would include epigenetic screening. The resulting "Faroes Statement," notable for its exigency, said, in part: "Toxicological tests and risk assessment of environmental chemicals need to take into account the susceptibility of early development and the long-term implications of adverse programming effects. Although test protocols exist to assess reproductive toxicity or developmental neurotoxicity, such tests are not routinely used, and the potential for such effects is therefore not necessarily considered in decisions on safety levels of environmental exposures."[45]

Among the health problems that might be better addressed if epigenetic screening was part of routine chemical testing were those Retha Newbold and her colleagues identified while investigating the impacts of DES. Among the possible epigenetic outcomes of chemical interference with endocrine hormones—or, in Theo Colborn's words, what these synthetic compounds can "mess up"—that Newbold's lab discovered was a misprogramming of how a body produces and stores fat. "Neonatal—or prenatal—exposure to estrogenic compounds alters body weight in animals," says Newbold of what she's observed in lab experiments. Her research has shown that mice exposed to DES during early stages of their development produced more and larger fat cells—a process called adipogenesis—and more abdominal fat, than those not exposed. Mice that were exposed became obese adults and remained obese even when they were put on reduced calorie and increased exercise regimes. Bruce Blumberg, a developmental and cell biologist at the University of California at Irvine, has dubbed these chemicals (there are a number that prompt adipogenesis, not just DES) "obesogens"—chemicals that prompt obesity.[46]

Blumberg began to suspect a link between chemical exposure and obesity when trying to pinpoint how another endocrine disrupter, the synthetic chemical called tributyltin, affects genetic mechanisms in the reproductive system. Not well known by name, tributyltin has been used as a marine and agricultural fungicide since the 1960s and 1970s. It's also been used as an antimicrobial agent in industrial water systems, livestock operations, and fish hatcheries. Tributyltin belongs to a class of compounds called organotins (constructed from tin and hydrocarbon molecules) that are readily absorbed by fish and shellfish.[47] Among its other applications are as a wood preservative, a glass coating, and as a stabilizer in silicones and plastics, including widely used polyvinyl chloride products. It has also been used to coat special baking and food preparation papers, but that was discontinued due to health concerns. And, notes a pesticide information bulletin published by a consortium of universities including UC Davis, Cornell, and Oregon State, "Evidence of organotins entering the human diet has been observed with Chinook salmon, which may be commercially raised in TBT [tributyltin]-treated pens."[48]

One of the most prevalent uses of tributyltin has been in anti-fouling paints on ships to discourage barnacles and algae. It inhibits the growth of marine life so successfully that it can essentially kill off lobster larvae and decimate oyster beds, as it did accidentally in France in the 1970s. Perhaps the most dramatic impact of tributyltin exposure, however, was the discovery in the 1970s and 1980s on the UK coast of gender-swapping or "imposex" snails—female snails that were growing male reproductive organs—an effect eventually traced to the snails' exposure to very small amounts of tributyltin.[49]

"Tributyltin was making female snails male and making male flounders female," Blumberg told me.[50] When he and his colleagues discovered a link between tributltin and obesity, it was accidental. They had set out to investigate how the compound was affecting sex determination in both vertebrates and invertebrates. Instead of discovering how tributyltin affected sex hormone receptors, Blumberg and colleagues found that it activated the nuclear hormone receptor responsible for maintaining the balance of fat cell production. "What we discovered," said Blumberg, "is that tributyltin disrupted the genetic interactions that regulate fat-cell activity in animals."

"Fat cells are an endocrine organ," explains Blumberg. And what he and his colleagues observed in animals exposed to tributyltin was remarkably similar to what Retha Newbold had observed resulting from DES exposure. "Exposure to tributyltin is increasing the number of fat cells, so the individual will get fatter faster as these cells produce more of the hormones that say 'feed me.'" Like DES, tributyltin appeared to permanently disrupt the hormonal mechanisms that regulate body weight. "It may not just be a matter of eating too much and exercising too little. You may come into this world with a programming set in motion by chemical exposure," explains Blumberg. "Once these genetic changes happen in utero, they are irreversible and with the individual for life," adds Newbold.

What happens is that the estrogen-like synthetic—be it DES, tributyltin, or another substance—interferes with the genetic receptors that determine the feedback loop between fat cells and the brain, Newbold told me. Instead of giving a signal that says, in effect, "Thank you very much, I've had enough to eat," these altered cells think they need more energy and so continue to demand food even when they've received enough nutrients. The result is an increase in the number of fat cells, the size of fat cells, and even locations of fat cells. Photographs of animals in Newbold's lab exposed to DES and those not exposed show striking differences. The exposed mice are plump dumplings and microscope slides of their tissues show large globular fat cells. Their unexposed cousins are lean and have distinctly smaller and more widely dispersed fat cells.

What's of potentially more concern even than these effects caused by DES and tributyltin is that similar fat-cell responses have been seen in animals exposed to bisphenol A. Frederick vom Saal's research indicates that exposure to low doses of bisphenol A, before or shortly after birth, can activate the genetic mechanisms that promote the kind of fat-cell activity Blumberg and Newbold saw in their experiments.[51] "These in utero effects are lifetime effects and they occur at phenomenally small levels" of exposure, says vom Saal. All of these scientists agree that many factors contribute to excess weight gain but mounting evidence suggests environmental chemical exposure is an important part of the mix, and given lifetime exposure to numerous chemicals with these potential impacts, it's something they believe must be investigated further. And fat cells, I learn, play a role that is far more important than being the physiological equivalent of a couch potato.

"Fat cells have hormone receptors," explains Tom Zoeller, a University of Massachusetts–Amherst biology professor whose research focuses on how endocrine hormones influence brain and nerve cell function. "The activity of those receptors can change the development of fat," and a synthetic chemical that can bind to these receptors might have the same effect," says Zoeller. The synthetic chemicals Bruce Blumberg, Retha Newbold, Frederick vom Saal, and their colleagues have been studying appear to have this ability: to affect how fat cells behave, influence the kind of signals they send the body, and where fat itself accumulates—all of which are important factors in overall health.

"Not that much attention has been paid to patterns of fat distribution. It's a very complicated issue. But estrogenic compounds like bisphenol A may affect fat distribution," Zoeller explains. This is significant because it's become increasingly apparent that where a person carries fat (and there are obvious difference between males and females) can have profound implications, particularly for cardiovascular and metabolic health. For example, excess abdominal fat is considered a predictor of the existence of abnormal insulin resistance, a condition that may put an individual at risk for developing diabetes. Bisphenol A, certain phthalates (a class of synthetic chemicals widely used in PVC and other consumer products), PCBs, dioxins, and chlorinated pesticides have all now been shown to disrupt how the body processes insulin—altering the biochemical balance in ways that can lead to diabetes and obesity.[52] Chemical exposure will not always cause these responses but if these genetic alterations take place at a crucial early stage in life, they will be with that individual permanently.

Zoeller goes on to explain that these synthetic chemicals have another route through which they can affect a body's metabolism and that is by interfering with thyroid hormones. Vital to the health of important bodily systems, among the roles of thyroid hormones are regulation of growth and metabolism and helping to control cardiovascular and reproductive systems. "PCBs, PBDEs, DES, and bisphenol A can all interact and bind with surprising affinity to thyroid hormone receptors," says Zoeller. This happens, in part, because these synthetic chemicals are structurally similar to naturally occurring hormones, including thyroid hormones (the phenol group plays a part here), enabling them to interact with these hormone receptors as two similarly shaped puzzle pieces might.

If a synthetic chemical finds its way to a thyroid hormone receptor instead of the hormone itself, it brings with it a different set of chemical elements than the body has evolved to expect and so gives the cell a misleading set of signals. Some synthetics, explains Zoeller, are able to bind with thyroid hormone receptors, but do not fit the binding sites perfectly, resulting in slight genetic damage that creates another possible disruption in hormones function. The resulting improper or mixed signals can set in motion a series of biochemical responses that may set the stage for future disease or health dysfunction.

This kind of disruption can affect not only how we process food, store energy, and bring new generations into the world, but also how our brains function. Thyroid and other endocrine hormones are vital to brain development, so anything that disrupts their activity can affect the nervous system, explains Zoeller. If a synthetic chemical such as bisphenol A binds to a thyroid hormone's estrogen receptors—which then bind to neurons—it has the potential to affect the cerebral cortex. If exposure occurs during fetal development, the outcome can have a lifelong impact. During the past decade a series of studies of both humans and animals have found that exposure to PCBs can lower IQ and increase the incidence of attention deficit disorder.[53] Such chemical exposure can also lead to increased risk for motor skills problems and degenerative nerve conditions like Parkinson's disease.[54]

As Zoeller and other investigators are learning, exposure to endocrine-disrupting chemicals can have an effect on neurological health throughout life. Exposure during early stages of development can create lifelong impacts but exposure later in life can also be significant. For example, in the past twenty years or so it's been discovered that, contrary to earlier assumptions, the mature brain does generate new nerve cells. Endocrine system hormones are essential to this process.[55]

Bernard Weiss, a professor of environmental medicine and pediatrics at the University of Rochester School of Medicine and Dentistry who studies the effects of environmental chemical exposure on the mature and aging brain, points out that while early development is a period of special sensitivity to toxic chemicals, late in life is "another period of enhanced vulnerability." At that point, he notes, "We are not as able as during earlier periods to compensate for toxic processes and many of our organ systems operate at diminished capacity. It is also a period when these reduced capacities may begin to reflect the damage inflicted earlier in life."[56] Research by Weiss and his colleagues indicates that interference with the hormones that keep a brain's regenerative and neural circulatory systems running smoothly later in life may lead to cognitive problems and may also be a factor in Alzheimer's and other neurological diseases. These environmental exposures and suite of impacts are now widespread enough to have become a matter of public health concern

✣ ✣ ✣

While bits of this science on these synthetic chemical health effects were finding their way to the general public in 2007 and 2008, members of a U.S. government science panel convened by the Department of Health and Human Services's National Toxicology Program (NTP) were meeting to assess the reproductive and developmental hazards posed by bisphenol A. Its determination will influence any future recommendation for restrictions on the use of BPA.

The NTP panel determined, in a report released in September 2008, that the compound does pose possible developmental, neurological, and reproductive health risks for fetuses, babies, young children, and those approaching puberty.[57] While this report is described as "final," it does not end the government review of BPA. Questions remain about the National Toxicology Program process itself, questions that are indicative of the problems inherent in current U.S. chemical regulatory process—and of how we've traditionally gone about creating synthetic materials.

Some of these problems came to light in the spring of 2007 when questions were raised about possible conflicts of interest posed by Sciences International, Inc., the for-profit organization that had been hired to conduct the NTP's bisphenol A study. Employees of that company, it was discovered, had also been advising chemical manufacturers, including Dow Chemical, a manufacturer of bisphenol A. After letters of objection from Senator Barbara Boxer and Representative Henry Waxman, both of California, and the nonprofit Environmental Working Group, the review process was temporarily halted.

Following this exchange, the National Institutes of Health (NIH)— the parent organization of the NTP—terminated its contract with Sciences International and the bisphenol A review panel convened without the company a month later. This panel, made up of about a dozen scientists who are not bisphenol A researchers, initially reached different conclusions from a separate panel convened by the NIH that included more than three dozen scientists who specialize in bisphenol A and endocrine-disrupter research. That second panel, which met in 2007, concluded that there is "great cause for concern with the potential for similar adverse effects in humans" as those seen in laboratory animals exposed to BPA.[58] This may seem like a bit of insider baseball—and it is, in a way— but it helps to understand why the official U.S. process for determining the regulation of a potentially harmful chemical used commercially is so cumbersome and often inconclusive.

Despite uncertainty about the full extent of potential adverse effects of bisphenol A on humans—and despite continuing safety assurances from the chemical and plastics industry as well as from government food safety agencies in the United States, Europe, and Japan—in the spring of 2008, a number of major North American retailers—including Wal-Mart, Toys "R" Us, and the CVS pharmacy chain—withdrew products for babies and children made with polycarbonate (of which bisphenol A is the key chemical ingredient) and are now offering alternative products.[59] At the same time, Health Canada, Canada's governmental health agency, announced a ban on BPA for baby bottles and placed the compound on Canada's toxic substance list.[60]

At about the same time in the spring of 2008, Nalgene—the manufacturer of refillable water bottles so widely used that the brand has become almost synonymous with the product—announced it would switch to a non-polycarbonate, non–bisphenol A–based plastic for many of these bottles. One of the materials Nalgene is using is a new polymer made by the Eastman Chemical Company. (Eastman also makes polycarbonate plastic, so clearly taking bisphenol A products off the market needn't sink a business.) But an investigation of information available on this new non–bisphenol A polymer, a product called Tritan, revealed the same assurances manufacturers have provided consumers for decades: The material is odor resistant and dishwasher- and microwave-safe.[61] It may indeed be entirely benign, but no data on environmental effects or toxicity are publicly available and we're still relying on a system that depends on manufacturers as the primary source for material safety information.

In response to a flurry of scientific journal publications and this growing public concern about bisphenol A, in April 2008 the U.S. Food and Drug Administration set up a task force to reevaluate the chemical's safety. Until this review is completed, the FDA says that current research indicates that "there is a large body of evidence that indicates that FDA-regulated products containing BPA currently on the market are safe and that exposure levels to BPA from food contact materials, including for infants and children, are below those that may cause health effects."[62] The European Food Safety Authority and Japanese National Institute of Advanced Industrial Science and Technology have come to similar conclusions.

The plastics industry similarly maintains that products made with bisphenol A pose no human health risks.[63] It does acknowledge that under certain conditions some polycarbonate products will degrade but assures consumers that visible wear does not indicate health hazards.[64] A chemical and plastics industry website called "Bisphenol-A.org" dismisses concerns about adverse health effects of bisphenol A exposure that might occur through normal use of polycarbonates by calling them "myths."[65]

Despite these assurances, as the number of scientific studies reporting adverse health effects of bisphenol A have proliferated, public concern about the chemical has grown. In response, a number of U.S. state legislatures introduced bills that would restrict the sale of products containing BPA—restrictions that focus primarily on products intended for children and infants—as well as other widely used synthetic chemicals that have also been identified as endocrine disruptors. As of this writing—in May 2009—only two bills restricting bisphenol A have yet passed, one in Minnesota and another in Chicago—in part because of vigorous lobbying on behalf of the plastics and chemical manufacturers.[66]

❖ ❖ ❖

Since 1997 well over 100 published studies have documented adverse effects in animals associated with exposure to low levels of bisphenol A. Theo Colborn and Frederic vom Saal note that studies that have found few or no health risks associated with bisphenol A examine potential effects at high rather than low doses and tend to be industry-funded. A *Washington Post* survey of bisphenol A studies conducted in 2008 found similar results on both counts.[67] Industry representatives counter that it's not a matter of keeping score of how many studies produce certain results, but a matter of scientific weight of evidence.

Weight of evidence typically means a decision based on the credibility of evidence. When evaluating health risks posed by exposure to airborne contaminants, the Environmental Protection Agency has suggested, the best evidence comes from human studies; when relying on animal studies, scientists must be satisfied that health effects in humans are likely to be the same as those in animals. (Interestingly, the genetic mechanisms involved in hormonal interactions related to bisphenol A, all the scientists I interviewed agreed, work the same way in all vertebrates.) The baseline for characterizing risk in such cases, writes the EPA, is how likely a substance is to cause cancer. If a substance is deemed carcinogenic, the EPA assumes no exposure is safe. But for non-cancer effects, the assumption is that there may be some level of exposure below which no ill effects occur.

When using such levels to set protective exposure standards, government regulations generally factor in a safety margin to allow for uncertainty and variations in response from individual to individual. "Long-term exposure to levels below these levels are assumed to produce no ill effects," writes the EPA.[68] This is precisely the dose-response assumption that endocrine disruption researchers say makes the current risk analysis–based system of chemical safety regulation that we now use inadequate to protect against chemicals that are biologically active at very low levels. And using acute carcinogenicity as a yardstick may not be the right measure when assessing a chemical's impact on the endocrine system, which may over time result in a suite of adverse health effects, including cancer.

Relying on carcinogenicity as the measure of a synthetic chemical's harm has resulted in some chemicals being deemed safe when in fact they have numerous potentially serious adverse impacts on how the body regulates and maintains health. Endocrine hormone research is relatively recent compared to cancer studies, but this information has now been with us for at least twenty years, and by continuing to omit these criteria our protection of public health from chemical hazards remains inadequate. This is one of the flaws in current chemical policy that adopting green chemistry principles could remedy.

Another problem with relying on the assumption that the higher the dose the more severe the impact is that it establishes as the norm what Joel Tickner of the University of Massachusetts School of Health and Environment calls "the never-ending discussion of 'how risky'"—endless discussions of what exposure level is safe.[69] (Such discussions have been going on for years around numerous synthetic chemicals—bisphenol A is now one, but trichloroethylene would be another example; lead exposure safety standards are another classic example of this problem.) These debates of "how risky" also tend to push the focus of safety discussions away from the environmental and health effects themselves and toward a conversation about statistics, risks, and benefits. The conversation often becomes one involving what have come to be called "stakeholders," parties with an interest—often a financial interest—in the outcome.

While poking around the various reports and commentaries on the recent bisphenol A review process I discovered that an organization called STATS[70]—a nonprofit associated with George Mason University with the stated aim of improving the quality of scientific and statistical information in public discourse—had posted a commentary about the 2007 *Washington Post* piece I had written on endocrine disruptors. It criticized the article for lack of what STATS called proper balance because the piece failed to include an independent view of the issues.[71] For such balance they recommended studies by the Harvard Center for Risk Analysis and the Gradient Corporation, an environmental consulting firm.

So I took a look. The Harvard Center for Risk Analysis's 2004 weight-of-evidence study on low-dose effects of bisphenol A was funded by the American Plastics Council and based its conclusions on nineteen studies.[72] The Gradient Corporation report, released in 2006, updated the Harvard Center for Risk Analysis study by reviewing an additional fifty studies.[73] It came to the same conclusion—that evidence does not consistently support adverse health effects resulting from low-dose exposure to bisphenol A. Both papers were published by peer-reviewed journals, just as the low-dose studies they criticize have been. The lead author on the Gradient study, however, has since testified before the Connecticut and Minnesota state legislatures on behalf of the American Chemistry Council in opposition to state bills that would restrict bisphenol A in children's products.[74] She has presented similar testimony to the Maryland state legislature—an effort a Maryland legislator described to the Associated Press as "heavy lobbying"—and also testified to the EPA on behalf of the American Petroleum Institute.[75]

Taking a closer look at STATS, I found that the organization describes itself as a "non-profit, nonpartisan research organization." A quick search into their background, however, reveals that they are affiliated with another nonprofit, the Center for Media and Public Affairs, that is funded by well-known partisan sources, including Richard M. Scaife and the John M. Olin Foundation.[76]

On the other side of the evidence aisle, in mid-2008 Theo Colborn and colleagues at the Endocrine Disruption Exchange—Colborn's nonprofit that studies environmental and health impacts of exposure to endocrine disrupting chemicals—had catalogued 335 low-dose studies of bisphenol A, of which some 81 percent found adverse effects at doses comparable to those included in the Harvard Center for Risk Analysis and Gradient studies.[77]

When it comes to protecting public or personal health, arguments about the significance of any adverse effects often come down to how one chooses to assess hazard and risk. Currently, our official chemical safety protocols have been based on determining "acceptable" levels of risk, the level of risk considered acceptable to achieve a particular benefit. This of course begs the question of "considered acceptable by whom." And it has generally rested on the premise that, in the absence of absolute proof of or any uncertainty about harm, there is safety. As we learn more about the subtle yet potentially profound effects that many of the numerous substances we're now routinely exposed to may have, this approach—prompted in part by consumers' concern—is beginning to change.

Nevertheless, a *New York Times* columnist, writing in the newspaper's science section in the summer of 2008, still dismissed concern over bisphenol A as a "myth," calling it an expensive health scare caused by a campaign led by a few researchers and activists, and saying definitively that "the dose makes the poison."[78] This misses the point by a wide mark, I think. All the scientists—researchers and medical doctors—I've queried on this subject agree that the findings of bisphenol A's adverse impacts have merit and demand further inquiry. All also agree that for the most potentially vulnerable human populations—infants; women who are pregnant, nursing, or planning to conceive; young children; or people with health conditions that would lead them to take special precautions— it might be wise to use alternatives to polycarbonates, since they are available. That the public has responded with such alacrity seems to me a reaction not to a "health scare," but a result of decades of being told various products were safe and without risk only to learn, in many cases too late, that they were not. Precaution has not gotten very good press in the United States, but given that we are now grappling with the results of what Alan Greenspan famously dubbed "irrational exuberance" in so many arenas—including the environmental—it's not surprising that with one small, controllable choice, so many people are choosing to err on the side of caution.

CHAPTER FIVE

Plasticizers
Health Risks or Fifty Years of Denial of Data?

"Children who live in homes with vinyl floors, which can emit phthalates, are twice as likely to have autism, according to a new study by Swedish and U.S. researchers." So ran the headline on a news story published on March 31, 2009.[1] While authors of this study called the findings "intriguing and baffling," the adverse health effects of phthalates—the chemicals used to make vinyl flexible and present in countless consumer products—have caused sufficient concern in recent years that in August 2008, the U.S. Congress, as part of a children's toy safety bill, decided to restrict the use of half a dozen phthalates in products intended for children under age twelve.[2] While chemical producers maintain that these compounds are safe, the same six phthalates have been barred from these and additional products in Europe since 2005 and Canada has had phthalate restrictions in place since 1998.[3]

Like bisphenol A, phthalates are used so extensively in so many products that most people encounter daily, items ranging from toys to toiletries, that our exposure to these synthetics has a similar potential to be continuous. And while they do not last long in the environment, these chemicals—which have been linked to reproductive and developmental abnormalities, among other endocrine system and health disorders—are so prevalent that as it has with bisphenol A, the U.S. Centers for Disease Control has found phthalates in the majority of Americans it has tested.[4] "Today there are no babies born without measurable levels of phthalates," says Shanna Swan, director of the Center for Reproductive Epidemiology at the University of Rochester School of Medicine and Dentistry, who's studied these compounds extensively.[5]

Phthalates are oily, colorless liquids—based on benzene chemistry—without which PVC (polyvinyl chloride) would be brittle and of limited use. Certain phthalates are used to create thin flexible films, lubricants, and solvents from various vinyl formulations that have both consumer and technical or industrial applications while others make fragrances last longer. There are at least two dozen different types of phthalates (chemically known as phthalate esters) with varying applications, varying molecular structures and, it's been discovered, varying biological activity and health impacts.

In one formulation or another, phthalates, either as plasticizers or fragrance agents, are used not only in toys (among them bath and teething toys) but also in upholstery, shower curtains, wire and cable coatings, car parts, food packaging (particularly coated paper and cardboard products[6]), medical equipment (medical tubing and IV bags, for example), the coatings of time-release medicines, shampoo, perfumes, insect repellants, and countless other products. Phthalates are also used in industrial and photographic film processes. The largest share of phthalates, however, goes into building and construction products—vinyl siding, window frames, doors, fencing, flooring, deck material, and piping (including water pipes)—to name but a few such products. In some bendable PVC products, phthalates can make up as much as 40 to 50 percent of the finished polymer. Over all, about 1 billion pounds or more are produced annually worldwide.

We take these chemicals into our bodies by ingesting them and by breathing them once their molecules have come detached from the materials they modify, and by absorbing them through our skin as we apply cosmetics, creams, lotions, and other skincare products. A study published in 2008 found that babies exposed to phthalates through lotions, powders, baby wipes, and shampoos had more phthalates in their urine than babies on whom these products were not used.[7] While phthalates are not environmentally persistent, there are enough of them escaping from products in the built environment that they're being found in waste-water, surface water, and in drinking water sources. But one of the main sources of concern for exposure are the phthalates used in plastic teething toys, vinyl bibs, pacifiers, and other items children chew and suck.

While parents and legislators are now turning to products without phthalates, the American Chemistry Council (ACC), an industry group, says their fears are ungrounded. "There is no reliable evidence that any phthalate has ever caused any harm to any human in their fifty-year history of use," says the ACC.

Yet numerous animal studies conducted since the 1970s indicate that certain phthalates can produce a suite of disturbing health effects—particularly on but not exclusively related to the reproductive system—including what some researchers call "phthalate syndrome." This series of health problems, prompted by insufficient androgen hormones (male sex hormones), results in effects that include reduced sperm production, increased risk of testicular cancer (now the most common cancer in young men), and the genital abnormalities that are currently the most common birth defects among American baby boys. (This condition, called hypospadias, the rate of which has doubled in the United States since 1970, is characterized by a defect in the penis that indicates reduced male characteristics.[8]) There's also evidence that certain phthalates' alteration of thyroid hormone and testosterone function can lead to metabolic disorders.[9] These compounds may be able to cross the placenta and influence the timing of labor.[10] Among the phthalate formulations that have been shown to have anti-androgenic or feminizing effects on male rats exposed just after birth, is one known as diisononyl phtalate or DINP. Exposure to DINP has also caused kidney and liver toxicity in adult mice and rats.[11] It is used in plastics and is now barred under the new U.S children's product safety bill. DINP is not bound into the plastic, so it can migrate into saliva and be swallowed if children mouth these products. "We're not yet sure what level of exposure produces these effects, but they are a real concern," says Paul Foster, senior toxicologist at the U.S. National Toxicology Program.[12]

Chemically, phthalates are hydrocarbon compounds made by varying the composition and structure of what's called benzenecarboxylic acid. Essentially they work by creating a chemical reaction that softens PVC and other polymers, including polyvinyl acetate, which is the base of many adhesives and glues and is also used in cosmetics. Phthalates can also be used as solvents for fragrances that will make the scents linger longer, a property that has made them ingredients of room deodorizers. They are used as lubricants and solvents in lotions. Phthalates make nail polish flexible enough to resist chipping. They enable pigment in mascara to form a flexible film, help eye shadow cling smoothly, and have been used in hairspray to keep the fixative from becoming too brittle. (The phthalate impacts, it should be noted, would be additional to and separate from those linked to the chemical components of vinyl chloride itself, which have been linked to liver and other cancers.[13])

Because there are so many different configurations of phthalates, these compounds are trickier to grapple with from a consumer and regulatory perspective than a single substance like bisphenol A. Apart from cosmetics, personal care, and some cleaning products, most items made with phthalates carry no ingredient labels. Food packaging, toys, tools, toothbrushes, and automotive parts are a few such products. And if phthalates are used in proprietary fragrance formulations, as they often are, a label will simply read "fragrance." Even if a product says it's made of PVC or contains polyvinyl acetate, the phthalate or phthalates used as plasticizers may not also be listed, making it hard for consumers to make independent choices about these chemicals.

As has often happened with U.S. environmental policy, American legislative efforts to curtail use of phthalates began in California. In 2006, San Francisco began prohibiting the six phthalates banned in Europe (these include DEHP, DINP and benzylbutyl phthalate, all used in PVC, as well as dibutyl phthalate, widely used in cosmetics) from toys and other products intended for children under three. The following year, the same substances were banned from comparable products throughout

California.[14] Since 2006—and in advance of any federal legislation—a number of other states have proposed similar restrictions, often in the company of bills that would also curtail use of bisphenol A and PBDE flame retardants.[15] The chemical industry has characterized such legislation as an overreaction to the risk posed by actual phthalate exposure, a response thus far echoed by both the U.S. Consumer Product Safety Commission and Food and Drug Administration.[16]

But moving ahead of the regulatory curve—and responding to consumer concern—many U.S. and international manufacturers, including Mattel, Procter & Gamble, L'Oréal, Nike, and Dell to name just a few, have already removed or are phasing out certain phthalates from various cosmetics, personal care, and infant products and are among the companies now offering phthalate-free sports gear, toys, cleaning products, and medical and electronic equipment. This, of course, makes good business sense. No one wants to be stuck with a line of products—a process—that is out of regulatory compliance or that the public is afraid to buy.

As has happened with other European hazardous materials restrictions—specifically regulations that curtail the use of certain toxic chemicals in electronics—the EU's restrictions on phthalates have spread to products destined for a wider international market. Since the EU ban of dibutyl phthalate (DBP) from cosmetics, for example, a number of major cosmetics manufacturers have removed the chemical from products sold internationally. Although these technical and tongue-twisting chemical names sound obscure, I knew this issue had reached the American mainstream when in the summer of 2007, my local newspaper's Sunday coupon inserts included one for Revlon nail polish that declared it "DBP-Free."

DBP-free nail polish may now be easy to find at the neighborhood drugstore, but another phthalate, diethylbutyl phthalate (DEP), is not yet restricted anywhere, although some U.S. state legislatures have proposed bills that would restrict its use. DEP is commonly used in personal care products, fragrances, and as a plasticizer as well as products that come into contact with food: treated papers, foils, and some of the clear plastics used as windows on bakery boxes. Food samples taken in the United

States and the UK have found DEP in baked goods—cakes, crackers, cookies—and candy, all presumed to have migrated from the packaging.[17] Since packaging typically carries no materials labeling, without regulation it's impossible to know if your candy bar might come with traces of phthalate.

Like other phthalates, DEP is easily absorbed through the skin and can be widely distributed through the body although it does not bio-accumulate, according to research published by the World Health Organization.[18] Human exposure, this research indicates, can be significant, occurring directly through the use of products containing DEP and environmentally from DEP that's entered air, water, and soil from waste, from manufacturing, and from products themselves. DEP has been found in wastewater in the United States, tap water in Japan, and in surface water in the United States, Canada, the UK, and various other European countries among other locations—ample evidence of its prevalence.

The U.S. Agency for Toxic Substances and Disease Registry (ATSDR) currently says there is no information about DEP's toxicity to humans who breathe, eat, or drink it. Yet according to the agency's website, "Some birth defects occurred in rats that received high doses of diethyl phthalate by injection during pregnancy." But, notes the ATSDR, "Humans are not exposed to diethyl phthalate by this route." So the significance of these findings is subject to debate.[19] In other phthalate studies, large doses of DBP (dibutyl phthalate) have caused tumors in lab rats and very large doses have lowered the quality of sperm produced.[20] Whether this can happen as a result of exposure to phthalates encountered environmentally is not known. Yet given that the reproductive system health problems being seen in people parallel the effects phthalates produce in animal studies, Paul Foster says he thinks these compounds are "really something to worry about."[21]

While manufacturers and consumers began to opt for products without phthalates, the Phthalates Esters Panel of the American Chemistry Council—an industry group made up of phthalate manufacturers including Eastman Chemical, BASF, Exxon Mobil, and the Ferro Corporation—continued to maintain that these compounds pose no human health risks and even asserted in a 2008 press conference that restrictions in the new U.S. children's product safety bill were "not based on science."[22]

"There is no scientific basis for Congress to restrict phthalates from toys and children's products. With over fifty years of research, phthalates are among the most thoroughly studied products in the world, and have been reviewed by multiple regulatory bodies in the U.S. and Europe," the American Chemistry Council announced in response to the 2008 legislation. The Phthalates Esters Panel media information kit, meanwhile, asserted that "there is no reliable evidence that any phthalate has ever caused any harm to anyone."[23] These and other bulletins issues by the American Chemistry Council claimed that there was insufficient evidence in any of the studies conducted thus far to infer that phthalates might cause any human reproductive health problems. In answer to the question, "Aren't phthalates endocrine disruptors?" the industry resource response was, "In lab tests with rodents, phthalates do not block the action of male or female hormones, or mimic their behavior."

Following the research into the behavior and health effects of commonly used phthalates, however, I found a somewhat different story. Concern about adverse effects of phthalates and their ability to migrate out of finished products seems to have burst onto the public scene in the United States only over the past several years, but it's been in scientific sights for more than forty years. The National Institutes of Health publication *Environmental Health Perspectives*, for example, devoted an entire issue to phthalate esters in 1973. The concerns raised then were of two kinds, not always related. One was concern over emerging evidence of phthalates' adverse health effects. The other was over the migration of phthalates from the plastics and polymers of which they were constituents and their ability to contaminate other substances—concerns that were discussed in the early 1960s.

In their introductory essay to that special issue, the editors pointed to the migration of phthalates into human blood in medical settings, with some nascent concerns about the resulting health effects. At that time phthalates had been found in both blood stored in PVC bags and in patients who'd received such blood in transfusions. Ten years later,

phthalate contamination of blood stored in PVC bags was discussed at a
1982 conference. But, given the inconclusive evidence about the precise
health effects of such exposure—including the then recently conducted
studies that indicated DEHP might be a carcinogen—this concern was
not shared with patients, "such as hemophiliacs and leukemics, whom we
feel are sufficiently burdened, and need not be concerned with question-
able numbers at this time," noted J. C. Fratanoni of the FDA's Division of
Blood and Blood Products.

Another paper published in 1973 based on studies done in Germany in
the 1960s found phthalates leaching out of PVC tubes used for milking.[24]
Concern about phthalates' tendency to migrate from PVC and other
polymers also came from researchers at the NASA Goddard Space Center
who were mainly interested in potential phthalate corruption of instru-
mentation, including sensitive mirrors and lenses. Space vessels, given
their enclosed environments, are by nature self-contaminating, and officials banned polyvinyl chlorides as a result. But PVC was so widely used
that phthalates were often found on spacecraft equipment or in these enclosed environments anyway as a result of PVC use in other equipment
involved in preparation of items destined for spacecraft—including the
air filters designed to remove contaminants.[25]

The degradation of polymers (and other materials) used on spacecraft
and submarines had already been a concern for a least a decade. In 1963,
the Aerospace Medical Division of the U.S. Air Force produced a report
examining the enclosed environment air-contamination potential of materials and their chemical constituents. This report noted the potential of
large fluorinated polymers, such as Teflon, to break down "into free radi-
cals which unzip into monomers," and of "hydrocarbon type polymers"
to "give off various hydrocarbon products of degradations such as methane, ethylene, and longer chain hydrocarbons." The authors also noted
that "polymers containing chlorine may evolve into hydrogen chloride
and possibly, phosgene." (The last concern, however, was focused on
degradation of the refrigerant Freon rather than of polymers.[26])

Forty years later, researchers at NASA released a white paper that discussed contamination of Mars landing vehicles by substances resulting

from polymer degradation and off-gassing—contamination from DEHP and other compounds that could interfere with the vehicles' measurement equipment.[27] I asked David Beaty, an author of the paper and chief scientist for NASA's Mars exploration program, about this. When searching for signals of life on Mars, it's important, Beaty explained, to be able to separate out "signal—if any—from noise." Therefore it's important for NASA scientists to know precisely which contaminants—including plasticizers—might migrate out of polymers, adhesive or coatings, for example, so that they can be taken out of the equation. Instrument function is also a concern, Beaty told me. It's not that phthalates themselves have caused problems, but that their migration is a reality that needs to be dealt with.

Even though NASA and others have recognized phthalate migration for decades, there is still resistance among industry trade groups. During a 2008 press teleconference held by the Phthalate Esters Panel of the American Chemistry Council, Dean Finney, a consultant with more than forty years experience working with phthalates, including thirty-eight years with Eastman Chemical, a manufacturer of phthalates, asserted without modification that phthalates "do not migrate" or "off gas."[28]

Because there are so many different types of phthalates, it's easy to become confused about which kinds are used in which products and, therefore, which compounds may be of particular concern in terms of human exposure. Bulletins issued by the Phthalates Ester Panel to defend phthalate safety have used this confusion to underscore lack of public understanding about these chemicals and to point to inaccuracies in reporting.[29] Yet adding to the complexity of phthalate behavior is the fact that once inside a human or other animal body these compounds break down into smaller—and, it turns out, biologically active—molecules known as metabolites. These are what will be present in blood and urine, so it's these phthalate metabolites, rather than the parent compounds, that the Centers for Disease Control has been measuring in its surveys of Americans' chemical exposures.

These metabolites are also what appear to be causing phthalates' observed health effects. As Paul Foster explains, while phthalates may at first be present in a mother-to-be (for example) in a nontoxic form, by the time her body has processed the compounds, they will likely be broken down into a reactive form that can then interact with her developing fetus. Further, as environmental health expert Dr. Ted Schettler told me, individual phthalate metabolites can cause different health effects.[30]

For example, a study published in 2007 found a link between a particular metabolite of DEHP—the most widely used PVC plasticizer—and altered thyroid hormone function.[31] (DEHP can also cause respiratory and immunological problems.) Another study, published in 2006, found that infants exposed to phthalates from PVC in medical equipment had concentrations of the resulting, biologically active metabolites in their urine, molecules that have been linked to adverse impacts on reproductive development.[32]

If these exposures take place very early in life, the changes produced by these chemicals can affect what Foster calls "primordial germ cells"— the cells that develop into eggs or sperm. These effects, he explains—like those induced by bisphenol A and the endocrine disruptors studied by Bruce Blumberg, Retha Newbold, and their colleagues—are permanent changes. This means that exposure before birth can prompt health effects that remain with an individual for life.

❖ ❖ ❖

Before delving further into how different phthalate metabolites behave, one way to begin thinking about or categorizing how different phthalates are used—and therefore how people may become exposed—is to understand that, generally, the physically bigger, heavier, formulations, including DEHP, are most often used with larger and bulkier materials like PVC. Molecularly lighter phthalates, including DBP (dibutyl benzyl phthalate), are used in more structurally delicate applications, such as adhesives or dyes, to lubricate textile fibers, in pesticides, and as part of the polyvinyl acetate emulsions used in glues, paints, and other coatings, including cosmetics.[33]

DEHP makes up about half of all such plasticizers used worldwide. In 2005, *Chemical & Engineering News* reported that about 300,000 tons were used annually in Europe.[34] U.S. production volume of DEHP, however, was a trade secret. Scores of studies undertaken since 2000 indicate that exposure to DEHP, especially before or shortly after birth, can adversely effect reproductive development, particularly in male infants. One source of such exposure is through medical equipment used in care of premature infants and developing embryos.[35]

Paul Foster points out that the male reproductive effects produced by DEHP and DBP exposure in humans can happen in the first or second trimester of pregnancy. This means it's entirely possible, he notes, that exposure to phthalates—or any other chemical that acts similarly—could take place before a woman might even be aware that she's pregnant, and therefore before she would have had a chance to take action to reduce her exposure. This also points again to the difficulty of relying on traditional toxicology to protect against chemical hazards: Here, timing of exposure may be as important a marker of toxicity as dose.

That many of the adverse health impacts of phthalates—like other endocrine disruptors—are subtle and do not fit into a direct cause-and-effect scenario makes them challenging to contend with from a regulatory perspective. That said, by the early 1970s, some rather dramatic changes had already been observed in lab animals exposed to phthalates. Research in 1973 at the University of Tennessee Medical Unit's Science Toxicology Laboratories noted that, compared to relevant control groups of research they had surveyed, "all of the PAEs [phthalic acid esters or phthalates] studies showed a deleterious effect upon the developing embryo and/or fetus. At one or more of the dose levels employed, some or all of the following effects were observed for each compound: resorptions [when the body or a cell absorbs a substance that it's losing, including an unviable fetus], gross abnormalities, skeletal malformations, fetal death, or decreased fetal size."[36] Abnormalities included lack of tail, twisted hind legs, and malformed ribs and skulls.

Researchers from the U.S. Food and Drug Administration followed up on these findings in 1982 with an assessment of the most toxic of the phthalates tested by the Tennessee researchers, dimethoxyethyl phthalate (DMEP), and found similarly toxic effects. The majority of rats exposed to DMEP in the early days of pregnancy produced fetuses with multiple malformations, among them serious defects in bone structure and the brain. Researchers also noted that phthalate exposure affected how the rats processed zinc, an element that appears to play a role in the development and behavior of male sex hormones.[37] The multiple congenital skeletal malformations resulting from this phthalate exposure prompted the study authors to make the comparison to thalidomide, a drug prescribed to pregnant women in the 1960s to treat morning sickness that resulted in severe birth defects, among them missing limbs.[38]

A specialty plasticizer, DMEP has been used in photographic compounds and various film applications. Xerox, Eastman Kodak, and Polaroid have held patents for products that might incorporate DMEP, while Eastman Kodak, Philip Morris, and others have also held patents that list DMEP as a component of cigarette filters. Although the compound is restricted in Europe, having been classified as toxic to reproduction by the European Commission, and also listed on the U.S. EPA's Toxic Substances Control Act Inventory (simply a list of chemicals used and produced commercially in the United States) since 1979, it is still manufactured and available for bulk purchase and therefore presumably still being used. Most of the manufacturers I found in a 2008 search were in China, but products made with DMEP have hit the world market, having been found in Australia in children's toys and exercise balls.[39]

In 1982, another U.S. government agency, the National Toxicology Program, that had been scrutinizing the health effects of three widely used phthalates—including DEHP—released the results of its investigation.[40] In that study DEHP was found to produce liver tumors in both rats and mice tested, and therefore was deemed a carcinogen—the official wording being that DEHP is "reasonably anticipated" to be carcinogenic to humans," a judgment also adopted by the EPA and Centers for Disease Control but still being debated both within the United States and internationally.[41] The Phthalates Esters Panel website does not include this health hazard information, however, but instead mentions that the U.S. Consumer Product Safety Commission does not consider another phthalate, DINP (used extensively in vinyl toys, including teething toys), to be a human carcinogen. More than twenty-five years after this National Toxicology Program assessment, and billions of pounds of phthalates later, the upshot is that in the United States—among other places—DEHP use is still largely unregulated.

In August 2008, following signing of the U.S. toy safety bill that restricts (but does not completely ban) six phthalates—including DEHP, DBP, and DINP but not DEP—from children's products, the Phthalate Esters Panel held a press conference to dispel concerns about the health impacts of these compounds. To do so, Ray David, a toxicologist with the BASF Corporation (an international chemicals manufacturer), pointed out flaws and uncertainties in several recent phthalate studies and emphasized the uncertainty of applying animal study results to people. "Phthalates are one of the most thoroughly tested families of compounds in use today," says the American Chemistry Council.[42] "No one," said David, "has come to any conclusion that phthalates are a risk for the human population."

❖ ❖ ❖

In the absence of definitive guidelines on materials like polycarbonates and phthalates, faced with conflicting information, and with so many studies showing adverse health effects, what's a consumer to do? The general stance from the American Chemistry Council is that the precautionary principle disregards science, but the advice from scientists I've spoken to is to be strategic and to make choices that have the greatest potential health benefits for you and your family.[43]

What that entails is open to interpretation. One can take a radical approach like Theo Colborn and eschew plastic containers altogether. "I put everything in glass," she told me. One can follow Fred vom Saal who says he never uses plastic dishes for hot food or in the microwave. Or one can take the specific pragmatic advice offered by such researchers as Patricia Hunt and Hugh Taylor.

"A primary route of exposure is ingestion," says Taylor of bisphenol A. So "bisphenol A is easy to avoid when pregnant. Don't eat canned goods, don't have dental sealants put in unless absolutely necessary, and use glass instead of plastic water bottles," he told me.[44] Hunt advises avoiding polycarbonate plastics when they become visibly rough—a sign of degradation that can indicate bisphenol A leaching (something the American Chemistry Council disputes).[45]

Although the presence of phthalates is trickier to avoid since they appear in so many variations—often completely without labeling—the scientists I spoke to advise a strategy similar to that suggested for protecting against bisphenol A exposure. Avoiding PVC products while pregnant—particularly in contact with food—can help prevent exposing a developing baby, says Shanna Swan. Like Swan, Paul Foster suggests that women who pregnant are or planning to become pregnant should take the most precautions.[46]

Not pregnant and not feeding a child, I've been wondering how finicky I should be about these compounds. The first time I heard about bisphenol A was at a lecture in 2005. After the talk, I went home and peered at the bottom of all my plastic containers, searching for a telltale sign indicating polycarbonate. (Typically this is a #7 or the word "other," but much polycarbonate is unlabeled.) I've since switched to stainless steel refillable water bottles and travel mugs and use a ceramic filter or glass to make coffee. And while I've never used plastic dishes or put plastic in a microwave, I've started to think twice about putting hot leftovers directly in any kind of plastic.

As for phthalates, I've become a ferocious reader of the tiny type on containers of anything I might use in the bathroom. I avoid anything that says "fragrance" and have learned that even "unscented" products often list "fragrance" as an ingredient. When it comes to vinyl, I won't choose it but I know there's PVC coated wiring in my house and attached to appliances. (Work is going on to design alternatives, but thus far non-PVC or other halogen-free coated wiring is not yet readily available for residential use, certainly not yet at a price that would challenge the PVC wiring now on the market.) At some point I'd like to replace the vinyl kitchen and bathroom flooring, but while I'm saving up to do that, I pay closer attention than ever before to what touches my food and skin, and I ask questions about anything new that comes into the house.

Still, a great many of the products that populate our lives carry no materials listings or have ingredients that require a major sleuthing expedition to discover—something most people are not prepared, willing, or even able to undertake. Often the people who are least likely to scan ingredient labels or to have considered these issues may be those whose circumstances make them particularly vulnerable to potential chemical hazards. This is true everywhere but particularly in less wealthy countries—and the latter often get overlooked in discussions of new and environmentally improved materials.

At the same time, not all products with the same ingredients listings are created equally well. One of the issues with materials that carry names like "vitamin E," for example, has to do with the compounds' source and production. There are vitamins, minerals, perfumes, and oils derived from naturally occurring sources and there are products with the same names that may be synthetics. Being a synthetic does not necessarily indicate a problem, but folks like those watchdogging the supply chain at the Environmental Working Group want to know where stuff comes from and how it was made before declaring it free of hazards. Given recent history with products as diverse as peanuts, milk, toy trains, pet food, and toothpaste, this seems to me a reasonable strategy.

❖ ❖ ❖

When it comes to a number of widely used, and therefore pervasive, mobile synthetics with adverse health impacts that are now well documented, the principle of precaution is slowly gaining ground in the United States. For example, independent of any regulation or legislation, as concern about the health effects of phthalates has grown, a number of hospitals have begun to move away from PVC products that contain DEHP. The organization Health Care Without Harm lists dozens of hospitals now doing so.[47] Health Care Without Harm also catalogues the PVC-free products now available for almost every hospital or medical use, from IV tubes, catheters, and blood bags to disposable gloves, flooring, cubicle materials, wall coverings, shower curtains, and office supplies. It's probably entirely unreasonable to avoid medical care for fear of phthalate exposure, but that there are hospitals using alternative products means, for example, that when available, one might be able to choose a PVC-free environment for obstetric and neonatal care. Meanwhile, the trade associations of the plastics manufacturers hold out hope that phthalates and bisphenol A will some day soon be given a clean bill of health.

Asked how to reconcile the blatantly contradictory statements coming from manufacturers of bisphenol A products, phthalates, and other so-called endocrine-disrupting chemicals and those coming from independent scientists, Shanna Swan utters the phrase "tobacco science." She cautions against consumer overreaction but points out that it was thirty years between the Surgeon General's Warning about cigarettes and the industry taking responsibility for tobacco's health impacts. Ted Schettler cautions against such a precise comparison because the modes of exposure differ so distinctly, but characterizes the chemical industry's stance on phthalates as "fifty years of complete denial of data."[48]

"Scientists never all agree," says Patricia Hunt. "There is always going to be controversy." Yet, she says, "If we wait it may be too late."

CHAPTER SIX

The Persistent and Pernicious

The village of Savoonga is perched on the edge of the Bering Sea just 150 miles south of the Arctic Circle. It sits on the north shore of Alaska's St. Lawrence Island, whose westernmost point—about 40 miles west of here—is only 40 miles from the Russian mainland. Low mountains rise east of the village, sloping up to the island's volcano. It's the third week of July 2007 and there is still snow on the higher ground. We are too far north for trees but the tundra is dotted with cottony blooms, tiny red sedum, shiny yellow buttercups, and violet gentians. When the clouds lift, the sky is a vibrant, cornflower blue. The sun will not set until after midnight.

There is no harbor here. The tundra stops at the short bluffs that rise just above the water. Whale vertebrae, ribs, and long strips of baleen are scattered along the shore. Fishing skiffs are pulled up onto the black sand and pebble beach on log rollers. Upturned umiak—the traditional, wood-framed Yup'ik boats—rest on tall sawhorses well above the water line. Supplies from the mainland—including fuel—arrive by barge or by air. Standing at the seaside cliffs north of town, where the tumble of boulders rustles with nesting murres and auklets as puffins ride the sunlit swells below, I find it's almost impossible to imagine that this Arctic island community is suffering the effects of persistent and pernicious industrial pollution.

I flew in from Nome under a low sky on a Bering Air flight with at least 200 cans of evaporated milk, cartons of diapers, one other passenger, and the pilot. A clutch of people—many of whom buzzed up the gravel road on ATVs, some pulling small cargo trailers—gathered to meet the plane. I traveled up from Anchorage with Viola Waghiyi, who coordinates the environmental health and justice program for the nonprofit Alaska Community Action on Toxics (ACAT). Savoonga is Vi's hometown, and it is through ACAT that the village's Tribal Council has granted me permission to visit so that I can attend meetings the U.S. Army Corps of Engineers is holding. They're here to discuss the latest phase in the cleanup of hundreds of thousands of gallons of toxic waste and contamination at the formerly used defense site at Northeast Cape, a place generations of St. Lawrence Island natives have used for hunting and fishing.[1]

Left behind when military operations closed here nearly forty years ago were PCBs, pesticides (among them mirex, used as both a flame retardant and pesticide and considered a probable human carcinogen), metals (including arsenic, chromium, and lead), brominated flame retardants, fuel oils, and various volatile organic compounds (solvents and degreasers)—substances that have now outlasted the military presence by decades.[2] There are more than 100 such sites of military contamination dotted across Alaska, most located in remote native communities.

In the early decades of the Cold War, communities along western Alaska's Norton Sound became sites for stations in what was called the Distance Early Warning System. Part of this system was a communications network known as White Alice, which consisted of huge enclosed transmission towers powered by diesel generators. They looked like a cross between Stonehenge and something designed for *2001: A Space Odyssey*. White Alice was in operation on St. Lawrence Island from the late 1950s until about 1972, by which time satellite communications had rendered it obsolete. One of the White Alice sites was at Northeast Cape, where from 1954 until 1972 the U.S. Air Force and Defense Department maintained a 4,800-acre surveillance and communications installation. The site included twenty-five industrial buildings along with runways, pipelines, waste sites, and housing for military personnel. When the military left, Vi tells me, "They left in the middle of the night. They left everything."

In 1971, when the Alaska Native Claims Settlement Act was passed, the two St. Lawrence Island villages, Savoonga and Gambell, opted out of the program in favor of owning their land. Now to visit either island village, one must have permission from the Tribal Council and without additional permission—plus a $100 "land-crossing" fee—nonresidents are not allowed outside the village boundaries. Savoonga has about 650 residents. They live in a cluster of small, one-story houses with tin roofs that sit on cement blocks for clearance above the tundra and volcanic gravel during winter snow and melt-season mud. Huge whale bones and wooden drying racks, now draped with long strips of salmon-pink seal meat, grace the front yards. A maze of aboveground pipes, many encased in long aluminum boxes, runs between the houses to connect them to the water and sewer system. In the new part of town, ATV-friendly pumice roads have replaced the boardwalks that wind between the village's older homes. Until the airstrip went in about thirty years ago, the only way from Savoonga to Gambell was by water or dog team. There are still plenty of dogs—woolly huskies—but four-wheelers and snow machines have eclipsed the sleds.

These are not the only changes that have taken place. "We used to have real ice here," Vi's brother tells me. "Two- to three-feet-high icebergs. They were a real blue color. Now the ice doesn't come anymore. It freezes here in December now, but ice used to come in October or even September," he tells me. "People want to come back," says Vi. "But they can't because of the pollution and the river fish—the salmon—are all gone."

What the Defense Department left behind at Northeast Cape included nearly 30,000 (55-gallon) barrels of discarded hazardous industrial fluids. While the base was in operation, huge amounts of diesel and other petroleum products were stored on site. In 1968 a spill sent 180,000 gallons of diesel and PCBs into the mouth of the Suqitugheneq River (called the Suqi for short), and another 500 gallons of fuel leaked when a pipeline broke in 1973. The first spill reportedly killed off the river's fish—salmon and Arctic char among them—a disaster from which the river is still recovering. When cleanup operations first got underway in the 1980s at Northeast Cape, the Army Corps of Engineers identified at least twenty-three sites requiring environmental investigation and 150 tons of soil and debris contaminated with metals, PCBs, petroleum, and other fuel oils. The military base structures were finally removed in 2003, but additional caches of toxic waste continue to be discovered in the area.[3]

Long before Northeast Cape became a U.S. military site, families spent the summer there fishing from the Suqi River, home to one of the island's most prolific fish runs; hunting reindeer; gathering greens and berries; and at sea, hunting seal, walrus, and whale. This was not recreational activity. Savoonga is a subsistence community. Its residents' health and well-being depend on what they harvest from the sea and land. "That's my garden. I eat from the sea there," Alex Akeya, one of the Yup'ik village elders, told me of Northeast Cape.

Families continued hunting, fishing, and gathering at Northeast Cape even after the military arrived. They built fishing camp cabins from wood salvaged from dumps at the base. Villagers describe the piles of cylinders and rusty barrels leaking fuel oil. They tell me about village men who worked on chemical and fuel clean ups without masks or other protective clothing and about families who had to be evacuated from fishing camps during the big oil spill.

Since the early 1990s, when the Army Corps of Engineers began actively investigating the chemical contamination at Northeast Cape, it's been discovered that residents of St. Lawrence Island have levels of PCBs in their blood considerably higher than the U.S. average. In fact, a study published in 2005 found the levels in Savoonga residents who spent time at Northeast Cape fishing and hunting camps to be six to nine times higher than average.[4] Subsequent studies found islanders to be carrying chlorinated pesticides in their blood, and fish and water taken from the

Suqi River, as well as plants and berries gathered nearby, are contaminated with PCBs. Whether or not these chemicals and the other contaminants at Northeast Cape are responsible for the cancers, miscarriages, tumors, and birth defects from which Savoonga residents have been suffering since the 1990s is very much a matter of debate among the government and other scientists monitoring the site. But the community of Savoonga considers the connection clear.

Part of what makes the debate now going on between Savoonga Island residents and the military and other government agencies so contentious is that PCBs and the other hazardous chemicals discarded at Northeast Cape are undeniably toxic, mobile, and long lasting. Of particular concern are the PCBs, pesticides, flame retardants, industrial solvents, and chemical compounds associated with fuel oils that belong to a class of chemicals known as halogenated aromatic hydrocarbons. Their molecular composition and structure has made them useful for squelching fires and preventing combustion, as well as for creating films, adhesives, polymers, and coatings in conjunction with other materials. These compounds' chemical constituents include hydrocarbon rings—the basic benzene molecule—and elements on the periodic table that belong to what's called the halogen group, such as bromine, chlorine, and fluorine. In addition to creating industrially useful substances, this chemical combination is also capable of biological activity in ways that can prompt certain cancers, interfere with healthy endocrine hormone behavior, and cause other adverse health effects including cardiovascular problems.[5]

Many halogenated hydrocarbons have been created intentionally, but this chemical combination is also a feature of dioxins—chlorinated compounds that are typically byproducts of manufacturing processes, among them those used to create pesticides, herbicides, and other chemicals; chlorine bleaching of paper pulp; and the burning of PVC plastics. The EPA considers dioxins "likely human carcinogens."[6] Incinerators, cement kilns, and coal-fired power plants can be a source of the dioxins that result from incomplete combustion. In addition to synthetic dioxins, there are also naturally occurring dioxins produced by forest fires, volcanoes, and wood burning. Synthetic and natural dioxins, however, have different chemical fingerprints and it's the synthetic dioxins that make up most of what's currently in the environment and that are of overwhelming concern.[7]

Dioxins and the chemicals that can behave comparably—which scientists sometimes refer to as "dioxin-like" because of similar molecular structure and/or because they carry traces of actual dioxins in their commercial mixtures—include PCBs (although to complicate matters, not all of the many PCB formulations are considered dioxins), Agent Orange (the defoliant used infamously during the Vietnam War), DDT and other chlorinated pesticides (including the mirex used at Northeast Cape), as well as certain perfluorinated and brominated compounds. There are so many sources of such compounds and they are so persistent that, according to the EPA, most people carry detectable levels of dioxins in their bodies. Linda Birnbaum, former head of the EPA's division of experimental toxicology and now director of the National Institute of Environmental Health Sciences, has called dioxin the most toxic manmade chemical.[8]

These compounds are so persistent, explains Birnbaum, that even when use of these substances is discontinued, these pollutants will likely be with us for the next twenty-five to fifty years. This is true of PCBs, DDT, and some other chlorinated pesticides that were taken out of use in the United States and many other countries in the 1970s, but this also looks to be the case for newer compounds including PBDEs (brominated flame retardants that bear striking structural similarities to PCBs). "Seventy percent of all PCBs are still somewhere in the environment," says Birnbaum.

There have been large-scale accidental releases of these chemicals— two of the best studied in terms of health and environmental impacts are the 1976 accident in Seveso, Italy, and the 1968 PCB contamination of rice oil that took place in Japan—and PCBs are present in a great many sites in the United States that qualify for cleanup under the federal Superfund program. But for the most part the dioxins and dioxin-like chemicals now present in the environment result from these substances' use in their intended applications and, in the case of PCBs, how they were disposed of after routine use.

According to the World Health Organization, over 90 percent of our exposure to dioxin comes from what we eat—mainly meat, dairy, fish, and shellfish, foods where these compounds have accumulated primarily in fat tissue. (The EPA puts this amount at over 95 percent.) These substances are fat-soluble and so lodge in fat tissue in plants and animals, climbing the food web as this energy is consumed and stored. The exposure that is likely to occur with each serving is probably very small, but given the great persistence of these compounds in the body, the amounts add up over time. According to the EPA, these small levels of dioxins can accumulate "over a lifetime and will persist for years, even if no additional exposure were to occur. This background exposure is likely to result in an increased risk of cancer and is uncomfortably close to levels that can cause subtle and adverse non-cancer effects in humans and animals."[9]

What makes assessments of the environmental and human health effects of dioxins and dioxin-like chemicals more complex is that we're now not dealing solely with legacy pollutants like PCBs. We're now trying to assess, notes Birnbaum, not just the impact of one set of such compounds or of a single substances (like DDT or Agent Orange), but the effects of "many other chemicals that look like and have impacts like dioxin." (Assessing the effects of mixtures of such chemicals—what is likely the reality for current environmental exposures—is only just beginning to be investigated.) Since we're all now exposed to least some of these compounds, the "real question we are faced with," says Birnbaum, "is are effects occurring in the general population today?"

For residents of Savoonga this is not a theoretical question. Among the many astonishing exchanges that I listen to in the course of the often tense and emotional meeting that July day in Savoonga is one in which the existence of globally mobile contaminants is used by government agency representatives to discount the effects of local pollution. "Northeast Cape is not the primary source of PCBs in this area," says Carey Cossaboom, project manager with the Army Corps of Engineers. "It's the global source. Levels here are no greater than in the Aleutian or the Canadian Arctic. You're eating the fish. You're eating the meat. It's the subsistence. I don't know what's causing the cancer but I don't believe it's Northeast Cape," he says.

The fact is, no matter where fingers are pointed, Savoonga residents are suffering a double, even triple whammy of persistent pollutant exposure. They live in the Arctic, the Northern Hemisphere's sink for long-lasting contaminants that swim, fly, and hop long distances—a process now being amplified by the effects of global warming. For a healthy diet they depend on marine mammals, fish, and other locally available animals (most of which are at the top of the fat-bearing food web and hence likely to carry the largest load of bioaccumulative chemicals). Add to this the military waste that has made St. Lawrence Island a potent local source of contaminants. And while it may seem a relatively trivial issue to those who live farther south, reliance on local foods is central to the culture and survival of native communities of the far north.

Research by Grace Egeland, Canada Research Chair in nutrition and health at McGill University, shows that traditional Arctic foods tend to provide more protein, vitamins, and minerals than typically available local market food, which is usually higher in carbohydrates, fat, and sugar. What I saw for sale in the Savoonga store—staples like flour, sugar, and coffee along with long-shelf-life processed and snack foods (all at exorbitant prices)—seemed to bear this out. Between worry about contaminants and changes in ice conditions and animal migration patterns that are altering when and where it's possible to hunt, residents of communities like Savoonga are being pushed away from the food that defines their home and culture. Consumption of readily available market foods has already begun to have adverse health impacts on Northern communities, among them conditions that can exacerbate or be exacerbated by some of the same health problems that endocrine-disrupting contaminants can cause.

Looking for human health effects, either in the general population or one as specific as that of Savoonga, has become more complex now that it's recognized that the dioxins and dioxin-like substances at issue here have endocrine-disrupting properties in addition to the carcinogenicity that initially marked them as toxic. "There's increasing concern about learning problems, immune system problems, asthma and allergies, autoimmune and cardiac diseases," that may be prompted by exposure to this class of chemicals, explains Linda Birnbaum. Pinpointing the causes of this array of health effects—along with reproductive and developmental problems—is often even more difficult than looking for precise causes of an acute disease like cancer. This detective work is further complicated by the fact that most of us are exposed to multiple chemicals throughout our lives—legacy contaminants like PCBs and chlorinated pesticides, along with shorter-lived contaminants like bisphenol A and phthalates, and the newer generation of persistent contaminants that include numerous synthetics used in products designed for our homes and offices, thus creating the potential for constant, close-proximity exposure.

❖ ❖ ❖

Among the chemicals that fall into this category of the potentially dioxin-like are another set of synthetic halogenated hydrocarbons that are both percolating through the atmosphere and wafting through indoor air: the brominated flame retardants known by their initials as PBDEs (polybrominated diphenyl ethers). These compounds, used extensively in numerous consumer products from textiles to electronics, have now been recognized as environmentally mobile as well: They become detached from and leave finished products and travel with air, water, and dust. Because they resist degradation they are also recognized as persistent contaminants and have now been linked to many disturbing health effects. Until about five years ago, PBDEs were barely known to anyone but those involved with monitoring environmental contaminants or who worked in industries that used the compounds—most notably manufacturers of upholstery, plastics, and the electronics that require flame-resistant plastic components. By 2005, however, it was hard to open a newspaper without finding a report of a local or regional study that documented evidence of PBDEs in people's blood, in breast milk, or in household dust.

In 2006, responding to the mounting concern about potential adverse health impacts, the European Union implemented restrictions on the use of several of these flame retardants in electrical equipment—restrictions that have been adopted by major electronics manufacturers as well as some furniture and other companies for their products sold worldwide. To date there is no comparable U.S. federal regulation but a number of individual states have adopted PBDE restrictions comparable to those now in effect in the EU, and U.S. production of some of these regulated compounds has been voluntarily discontinued. Washington state and Maine have restricted all commonly used PBDEs, while many other states are considering such legislation. But PBDEs are not the only brominated flame retardants and altogether these compounds continue to be used at enormous volume despite restrictions.

Brominated flame retardants (or BFRs as they are sometimes called) work because the bromine literally retards the spread of fire by using up the available oxygen before it can fan the flames. Because bromine is readily available and these compounds work well with a variety of plastics and textiles, BFRs have been a cost-effective way to meet fire-resistance standards, particularly for furniture and electronics. Exact amounts produced are hard to get at, but one industry estimate put the 2001 world market for BFRs at 200,000 tons. With plastics, these bromine compounds are used as additives. This is an important point for understanding how these compounds escape the products they were meant to protect. They are not molecularly bound into the base material—the plastic—but are dropped into the mixture as one might drop a handful of chopped herbs into a batch of scrambled eggs, which means it's possible for them at some point to become detached.

PBDEs have been in commercial use at high volume since the 1970s. Some of the initial research investigating the effects of brominated flame retardants came in the 1980s and 1990s, when PBDEs started being detected in the environment in northern Europe. By the late 1990s and 2000, levels being measured in breast milk were increasing twofold every five years.[10] Shortly thereafter, it was found that the levels of PBDEs in San Francisco Bay harbor seals had increased one hundredfold between 1988 and 2000. Studies by Ronald Hites and his colleagues at the University of Indiana published in 2004 found that levels of PBDEs in people had increased by a factor of 100 since the 1970s, with levels in younger people and children higher than those in older people.[11] As more and more such studies found disconcertingly high levels of PBDEs in U.S. families—and in remote locations in the Arctic—concern about the compounds' persistence and potential impacts grew quickly.

In 2002 and 2003, brominated flame retardant producers, however, were distributing literature that claimed PBDE did not resemble PCBs and were most likely present in the environment as a result of their use in hydraulic drilling fluid in the 1980s. The Bromine Science and Environment Forum (BSEF) website—the organization of bromine product manufacturers—includes in its information about BFRs the following question and elusive answer: "Can brominated flame retardants be released from consumer products?" BSEF: "All studies confirmed that consumer exposure from BFRs is negligible."[12]

This stands in marked contrast to the reams of studies now published measuring PBDEs in household dust from both surfaces and vacuum cleaners, in dryer lint, in toddlers' blood, and in groceries. PBDEs have been gathered by wiping surfaces of computer cases with a filter paper dipped in solvent. The Arctic Monitoring and Assessment Program (AMAP) has found PBDEs in the Arctic—including the Alaskan Arctic—where levels of all brominated flame retardants have been increasing since 2002. Brominated flame retardants have now been found in sperm whales that cruise the deep ocean, in dolphins in the Gulf of Mexico, in China's Pearl River Delta, and in cheese, ice cream, and cat food purchased in the United States, as well as in the majority of Americans tested by the Centers for Disease Control.

Essentially, everywhere scientists have looked for brominated flame retardants, they have found them. Not surprisingly, very high levels have been found in China among workers dismantling electronics and in children who live and work at a dump site in Nicaragua. But they've also been found in children in middle-class California homes, in nursing mothers in the U.S. Pacific Northwest and, to a lesser extent, in people from all walks of life across Europe, as well as in food purchased across the United States, in polar bears and gulls, and in salmon both farmed and wild. Arnold Schecter, professor of environmental sciences at the University of

Texas School of Public Health, and his colleagues have been testing different indoor air environments and foodstuffs for the presence of PBDEs. New homes in the Dallas area with new carpeting had much higher levels than older houses tested. Air inside cars (brominated flame retardants are used in car upholstery and plastics) was notably higher than that in outside air. And confirming the fact that PBDEs are soluble in and have an affinity for fat, Professor Schecter's lab found that a Pizza Hut pizza had higher PBDE levels than vegetables, but even the veggie burger ordered from Burger King they tested contained some PBDEs.[13] Clearly, these compounds are nearly everywhere and we're eating and breathing them regularly.

So what are these compounds doing once inside of us? It's now generally accepted in the scientific community that PBDEs can interfere with endocrine hormone function and in doing so disrupt the normal workings of thyroid hormones. In animals, PBDEs have been documented to interfere with genetic receptors that trigger the release of the hormones that regulate reproductive development. They appear to affect both estrogen and androgen function, thus having a potential impact on the timing of puberty and both male and female reproductive health. In laboratory rats, certain PBDE molecules also affect neurological development and adversely impact sensory and cognitive function. PBDEs have also been shown to cause liver and immune system toxicity. If the exposure happens at a precise point in early brain development these effects—like those of comparably timed exposure to other endocrine disruptors—appear to be permanent.

However, not all brominated flame retardants or even all PBDEs behave in the same way. Generally, polybrominated diphenyl ethers have been used commercially in formulations of penta-, octa-, and decabromodiphenyl ethers, each named for the number of bromine atoms involved. Given its large, ten-bromine size, deca-BDE was assumed to be a more stable compound than the other commercial PBDE formulations with fewer bromines, and therefore to be an inherently less reactive and safer material. Because of their relative instability, penta- and octa-BDE (used in electronics as well as in upholstery foam and textiles) were re-stricted by EU regulations that went into effect in 2006. In 2004, following numerous studies indicating their persistence and potential toxicity, penta- and octa-BDE were voluntarily discontinued by their U.S. manu-facturers. (Of course, products made with these compounds are still around, both in use and in disposal sites, all around the world.) Despite the presumed stability and therefore safety of deca-BDE, it has produced some tumor activity in animal studies so the EPA has now classified deca-BDE as a possible human carcinogen.[14] Yet deca-BDE remains largely un-regulated. Nevertheless, manufacturers have begun to move away from this compound either in favor of other brominated flame retardants (al-ternatives that turn out to have their own environmental and health prob-lems, many similar to those of PBDEs) or are redesigning products to eliminate the need for brominated flame retardants altogether.

Since deca-BDE is the PBDE now in greatest use, a big question now being investigated from various perspectives is whether deca-BDE breaks down into smaller, more biologically active molecules once in the envi-ronment. The smaller PBDEs—those with fewer bromine molecules (like penta- or octa-BDE)—appear to be more readily absorbed by fat tissue and therefore to have greater potential to create adverse health effects than the larger compounds. While there are three or four predominant commercial formulations of PBDEs, there are actually 209 different con-figurations—or cogeners—of the PBDE molecule, and combinations of those 209 make up the commercial mixtures. These 209 members of the PBDE family are what scientists have been identifying when they mea-sure PBDEs outside of consumer products. Each of the 209 have specific characteristics that can help trace errant PBDE molecules from where they've ended up in living cells back to their sources in finished products. These traits also provide clues to the chemicals' behavior.

While the spotlight has been on the potentially adverse health effects of PBDEs, prompting manufacturers to seek alternative flame retardants, worrisome environmental and health information about some of these other products has also begun to emerge. It also offers a good lesson in how substituting one synthetic chemical for another—without asking the kind of questions green chemistry requires—will not necessarily result in improvements in environmental health or safety.

Among the non-PBDE brominated flame retardants commonly used in plastics—including consumer electronics—is one with the polysyllabic name of hexabromocyclododecane (HBCD). This flame retardant has thus far been used at less volume than PBDEs but as the latter have been restricted and withdrawn, use of HBCD has increased, especially in Europe where it's now the second highest flame retardant sold by volume. It's currently used in polystyrene, upholstery textiles, molded insulation, and hard plastics destined for construction and electronics among other products. Consequently, HBCD is now prevalent enough for scientists to refer to it as "ubiquitous."

Like PBDEs, HBCD is an additive flame retardant, meaning it's mixed into rather than chemically bound to the material it's intended to protect. While HBCD is now undergoing governmental risk assessments, its use is now unrestricted. The result of one such study, issued by the European Commission in May 2008, offers a confusing assessment by describing HBCD as persistent, bioaccumulative, and toxic, but also citing studies that found the compound degrading more quickly than previously thought.

From a green chemistry point of view, however, HBCD bears many similarities to the PBDEs it may be replacing. Like PBDEs it is fat-soluble and thus has been detected in fatty marine animals including dophins and porpoises, as well as in fish, breast milk, and umbilical cord serum. Like PBDEs, it has been found in indoor dust and human blood. The highest concentrations found thus far have been in top predators and birds of prey, leading researchers to suspect that it is working its way up the food web and in the process becoming more concentrated.[15] It is swirling around the North Sea, has been discovered in river sediment in Sweden, and has now been found in many places in the Arctic.[16] HBCD seems to travel by both air and water, putting it in the category of Frank Wania's hoppers—molecules that both swim and fly, hopscotching their way around the globe. A study published in April 2009 found that exposure to

HBCD led kestrels to lay eggs with thinner shells, have fewer chicks, and reproduce less successfully than birds not exposed, leading researchers to make the comparison to the effects of DDT on raptors—a chemical exposure that led to a decline of eagles and peregrine falcons.[17]

HBCD is less well studied than PBDEs, but thus far the effects associated with animal studies are similar. Like PBDEs, HBCD appears to interfere with endocrine hormones, including thyroid hormones, and has been observed to cause learning and memory defects in mice that were exposed to the compound shortly after birth.[18] One study published in April 2008 found that HBCD affected liver cells where, depending on the sex of the animal exposed, the compound then affected the behavior of either genes that influence thyroid hormone production, cholesterol levels, or the processing of fat.[19] What complicates the study of HBCD's health effects is that the compound exists in different structural forms called isomers. These varying configurations determine the compound's physical mobility and biological activity. Certain isomers appear to be more easily metabolized, detoxified, and excreted than others. In a confirmation of its dioxin-like characteristics, one of the HBCD isomers appears to interact with a particular enzyme present in animal cell nuclei that is associated with dioxins. When activated, this enzyme can respond in a way that triggers dysfunctional hormone signals. These observations led Linda Birnbaum to remark, "This compound frankly scares the heck out of me. . . . Why we would [consider HBCD as an environmentally acceptable alternative to PBDEs] is confusing."[20]

While these PBDEs, other halogenated hydrocarbons, and dioxin-like synthetic compounds are traveling enormous distances, research to determine how they affect living cells is taking place on an infinitesimal scale. Scientists are now trying to determine how these chemicals interact with individual genetic receptors, for it is at this level that such foreign substances apparently prompt cellular activity to go awry. Genetic receptors are specific sites on individual genes in a cell's nucleus to which specific hormones and other cellular materials, typically proteins and enzymes, bind. This coupling—picture jigsaw puzzle pieces coming together—will then prompt a biochemical reaction that sets in motion a chain of physiological and biochemical events that can determine the activity, and therefore the health, of a whole suite of bodily systems. And it turns out that there is a specific genetic receptor with which dioxin and dioxin-like chemicals interact.

John Stegeman, a senior scientist emeritus at the Woods Hole Oceanographic Institution (WHOI) and the director of WHOI's Center for Ocean and Human Health, explained this process to me patiently and with diagrams on the blackboard. What happens, he said—drawing a circle to represent a cell's nucleus and an arrow to show the incoming foreign object—is that when a xenobiotic substance, likely a toxin (but it might also be a drug), enters the body, certain genetic receptors react by releasing a special protein. In the case of dioxin or a dioxin-like compound, this protein is likely to be an enzyme in the family of enzymes called cytochrome P450. If the alien substance is dioxin, the enzyme released will most likely be one that's been labeled P450 1A1. When the dioxin—typically traveling in tandem with a larger molecular structure called a ligand that influences how and where molecules bind—reaches the key genetic receptor, the interaction between this biochemical newcomer and the receptor prompts a specific bit of DNA to send a message to an equally specific bit of RNA. This signaling process is called transcription, and what the DNA is telling the RNA here is to release cytochrome P450 1A1.

This family of enzymes, which exists in all animals, plays many vital roles. These enzymes are involved with metabolism, fat and hormone production, and responding to foreign substances, whether toxins or pharmaceuticals. The liver, not surprisingly given its role in coping with toxins, is home to many of these enzymes, some of which function specifically as detoxifying agents. When dioxin enters the picture, it interferes with the normal function of the AhR receptor, the key receptor with which halogenated hydrocarbons are associated. This interference can throw the body's enzyme production off balance. Because this disruption can affect everything from endocrine-system hormones and enzymes that process iron in blood and deal with calcium and cholesterol, to those involved with immune and nervous system function, the potential range of effects is large. For example, if AhR receptors in the female reproductive system are affected, the suite of hormonal reactions that trigger and regulate egg cell production can be altered. It's thought that the interaction between dioxins and these genetic receptors may also be involved in both promoting and suppressing growth of certain tumors and in determining reproductive mechanisms that can result in birth defects. It also appears that the genetic transcriptions prompted by this chemical signaling can alter a body's response to various chemicals and may influence how an individual responds when exposed to a carcinogen. Some of these chemical sensitivities can even be transcribed into genes in ways that enable them to be passed on to a subsequent generation.

As scientists continue to gather information on the environmental and health effects of PBDEs and HBCD, another brominated flame retardant widely used in electronics, tetrabromobisphenol A (TBBPA), has come under scrutiny. Tetrabromobisphenol A has also been found to accumulate in fat tissue and have adverse impacts on endocrine system hormones, liver and kidney cells, and the nervous system.[21] One of TBBPA's breakdown products is bisphenol A, raising the suite of concerns associated with that compound. As evidence of this set of flame retardants' toxicity accumulates, manufacturers are beginning to shift to alternative products.

At the same time, some industries that have used brominated flame retardants extensively in their products have begun to redesign them to avoid the need for these additives. Electronics manufacturers, among them Apple, Dell, HP, and Lenovo, are now phasing out the use of brominated flame retardants altogether. These manufacturers are also phasing out PVC, a move that reduces potential phthalate exposure and the possibility of the PVC releasing dioxins in disposal or if burned. In one example of redesign to eliminate BFRs, some Apple laptops and other products are now being made with aluminum cases rather than the kinds of plastics that need BFRs to meet fire-safety standards.

The concern always remains that making one change to reduce an adverse environmental or footprint impact may create a new and different impact and expand that footprint elsewhere. Simply substituting a new material with a particular function for another may not actually eliminate hazards, particularly under our current chemical regulatory scheme. What's happening with brominated flame retardants is an excellent example.

When the PBDE with five bromines (pentabromodiphenyl ether) was taken off the market in response to concerns about its biological activity and toxicity, a new brominated flame retardant (with the tradename Firemaster 550) was introduced to take its place, particularly in polyurethane upholstery foam where penta- was used extensively. Produced commercially since 2004 by the same company that was the sole U.S. manufacturer of penta-BDE (and that produced polybrominated biphenyls, the now-banned precursors to penta-), Firemaster 550 is now the flame retardant used most widely in products sold in California, a state that would by itself qualify as the world's eighth-largest economy, just to give a sense of the volume.

The precise chemical formulation of Firemaster 550 is proprietary information. But it's a brominated compound formulated with triphenyl phosphate—another flame retardant produced at high volume (at more than 1 million pounds annually in the United States), known to cause allergic reactions in people and be toxic to fish and other aquatic organisms.[22] The Material Safety Data Sheet for Firemaster 550—information provided by the manufacturer and currently the only publicly available environmental or health information about the product—leaves many gaps. It does, however, acknowledge that the compound is toxic to aquatic organisms and should not be released to water. It also reports that ingestion may cause nervous system effects, as may inhalation. "Long term oral overexposure," notes the safety sheet, "may cause kidney damage based on animal data. Prolonged or repeated exposure may cause liver, adrenal, thymus, reproductive, developmental, and neurological effects based on animal data."[23] Nevertheless, Firemaster 550's manufacturer told *Chemical & Engineering News* in 2003 that the compound has been given "a clean bill of health" in third-party testing by the EPA for persistence, bioaccumulation, and toxicity.[24]

Firemaster 550 has since been found in biosolids (a nice name for sewage sludge) collected at municipal treatment plants that discharge into San Francisco Bay and in household dust samples collected in New England. The scientists who analyzed the biosolid samples identified one of the chemicals detected in Firemaster 550 as tetrabromophthalate— a brominated phthalate and yet another halogenated hydrocarbon— of which millions of pounds are used annually the United States as a plasticizer for PVC, as wire insulation, and as fabric coating among other applications.[25]

In 2008, after Firemaster 550 was discovered in California wastewater treatment plant samples, its manufacturer, Chemtura, issued a statement saying that it had "evaluated the bromine component of Firemaster 550 in accordance with EPA guidance for toxicity and submitted the data for the EPA to review," and had not "fully commercialized" Firemaster 550 until the EPA had completed its assessment.[26]

Assuming Chemtura's statements about Firemaster 550 are accurate, clearly something is amiss with our chemical safety process if a new synthetic material can be given commercial go-ahead despite environmental persistence and evidence of toxicity to aquatic organisms, let alone similarity to other compounds with known adverse health effects. It also seems clear that simply adding new substances to lists of those we've banned or restricted—without addressing what makes them toxic—is not an effective way of keeping comparable materials out of production.

❖ ❖ ❖

"Why weren't we asking the right questions? Why didn't we have the knowledge of why something is toxic?" Paul Anastas asks rhetorically when I speak to him in his office at Yale University, where he heads the Center for Green Chemistry and Engineering. "No one has been asking to make [the] reduction of hazard a performance criterion. We have to change the idea of environment as a constraint to performance and make it part of design criteria."

It's a sunny, warm October day in 2007 when I visit Anastas in New Haven, and Yale is in the midst of a renovation boom. Construction is going on everywhere, including at the Sterling Chemistry building, a gloomy, medieval-looking building that he calls "Hogwarts." Anastas is approachable, very personable, and visibly excited about his work. His face lights up when he begins to answer my questions. He has a gently forceful and exceptionally clear way of speaking that I imagine was honed during his years in Washington, working with the Environmental Protection Agency, where he served as chief of the industrial chemistry branch from 1989 to 1998 before becoming assistant director for environment in the White House Office of Science and Technology Policy, a post he held from 1999 to 2004. In addition to teaching and working on policy, Anastas also works with businesses on green chemistry issues.

"I tend to be on the solutions side of things," Anastas tells me. "We don't just need to make people afraid, we need to get toxics out of our bodies and out of our newborns," his conviction clearly is amplified by the pleasure he takes in telling me he's recently become a father for the first time. "We need to know if a new material is safe or if it can be made safe."

So how do we do that? I ask.

To begin with, says Anastas, we need to be asking a whole series of questions that we simply haven't been asking while designing new materials. "Is it hazardous? What is its biological activity? What does the substance do to a body and what does the body do to the substance? Can it get into the body?" If so, what happens then? How is it absorbed and metabolized? What organs might it target? Can it cross biological membranes or the blood-brain barrier? Is the substance persistent and will it bioaccumulate? These are the questions Anastas and John Warner have incorporated into their principles of green chemistry. And they are essential to the narrative Warner is so passionate about bringing back to the science of creating new materials.

Answering these questions, Anastas explains, means looking at a substance's fundamental physical characteristics, beginning with its solubility. Solubility is important because whether a substance is soluble in water or fat determines how persistent a substance will be. A substance that is soluble in fat will tend to find its way into plant and animal cells where it may interact chemically with other cellular materials. If that plant or animal is a food source, then that fat-soluble substance can then begin its climb up the food web. (This is precisely what's been happening with the PCBs, PBDEs, and other persistent pollutants in the Arctic.) Water-soluble substances are less likely to bioaccumulate and more likely to break down swiftly in the world's—and the human body's—watery environment.

Anastas reminds me that one of the fundamentals of commercially manufactured materials as they have been produced throughout history is performance. This—along with upfront production costs and speed to market—has been the overriding characteristic by which the success of new materials has been measured. (PCBs do their job. So do chlorinated pesticides.) To change this pattern, says Anastas, "We need to characterize materials in terms of human health and the environment."

"We also have to get business to change," Anastas continues. "Ultimately it will be the cost factor. It will be more profitable to do it another way than we are now, so that we'll have to spend less on waste management and worker protection," he says. "There's a business case to be made for green chemistry, if only from an efficiency standpoint." As he says this I think about the enormous costs—financial, environmental, and human—involved with chemical waste on St. Lawrence Island. "What will it take to make green chemistry the norm?" I ask.

Part of what needs to happen, says Anastas is that "entrenched capital processes will have to be displaced." We have a long history with the suite of materials we are now using, with considerable investment of capital and infrastructure—and considerable profits in both. (The generations of brominated and chlorinated hydrocarbons fit this pattern.) To make the design changes in synthetics that need to happen, we need to work at the very beginning—the materials origins—of the supply chain. "If you address sustainability in unsustainable ways, you haven't done anyone any favors," says Anastas. "Green chemistry," he reminds me, "is not just a list of things that aren't allowed or what you can't do. We need to look at types of intrinsic hazards. . . . It comes down to the basics of molecular design." Again I think this is exactly what has *not* been considered in the design of PBDEs and other brominated flame retardants.

"Right now, our way of reducing hazard is all geared to lowering exposure to hazardous substances. [But] smokestacks, respirators, scrubbers, gloves—they fail and break. These technologies are a cost drain and can't add value efficiency or performance capabilities to a product.

Incremental improvement is essential but we need to have whole-system thinking," says Anastas.

"The regulatory pathway over the past twenty years is completely tied up in knots," he says. And the framework on which regulation now rests—bans and regulations to reduce exposure to hazards—won't result in change at the pace it urgently needs to happen, he tells me.

❖ ❖ ❖

The fact that so many compounds based on molecular structures with intrinsic environmental and health hazards are now virtually omnipresent throughout our lives—often beginning before birth—increases the chances that our cells will, at some point, be dealing with them. We now know that PCBs, chlorinated pesticides, numerous brominated flame retardants, and other synthetic chemicals with comparable chemical compositions and structures—all halogenated hydrocarbons—interact with genetic mechanisms that are present in all vertebrates. That they do makes it plausible to extrapolate from effects observed in animals—in the laboratory or field—to those that may occur in humans. Yet precisely how these impacts will manifest themselves—and in whom—is much more difficult to predict. Exposure to these compounds will not prompt the same response in all individuals, and some individuals may not experience any evidence of adverse response.

From this unpredictability stems the frustration—and fear—with which people like the residents of Savoonga are coping. The Army Corps of Engineers has advocated a cleanup plan for Northeast Cape that would leave fuel oil, PCBs, and other persistent industrial chemical contamination—flame retardants, pesticides, and solvents—behind to dissipate over time. "What scares me today is the scale and magnitude of the destruction," says Delbert Pungowiyi, president of the Savoonga Tribal Council, referring to the extent of pollution caused by the military base at Northeast Cape. "We've been put at risk for too long. We've been contaminated and it looks like we're being asked to take a chance again."

"We have a mission and it's black and white," said Carey Cossaboom of the Army Corps of Engineers at the meeting in Savoonga. "My mission is not to deal with the unknown," he says as one community member after another speaks of their own and family members' grave illness.

Linking a particular environmental chemical exposure to a specific person's illness is rarely a black-and-white issue, however. There will nearly always be unknowns. What is known, though, is that the military materials left behind at Northeast Cape are persistent and can last for decades. It is also now well documented that the chemistry of these materials makes them biologically active and extremely toxic.

We also now know that despite this evidence and knowledge, subsequent generations of synthetic materials based on comparable chemistry have been launched into commercial production for use in the consumer products that now populate our lives. This is precisely the knowledge on which green chemistry is asking those who design and manufacture new materials to act, so we can prevent the creation of yet more synthetic chemicals persistent and pernicious enough to disrupt—not just an individual's health—but the fabric of life for entire communities as they have in Savoonga.

CHAPTER SEVEN

Out of the Frying Pan

How could we as a society produce and use such large quantities of what were once "laboratory curiosities" with so few questions asked and such limited knowledge of the environmental fate of so many of these materials? And how is it that we have now launched into the world's atmosphere and the innermost workings of our biological lives so many engineered materials that seem to be interfering with the most fundamental biochemical processes of life—whether as endocrine disruptors or other inducers of cellular dysfunction? One place to start to understand how we've arrived at this point is by recognizing that historically, as illustrated by synthetics like bisphenol A, to assess the safety of commercially manufactured chemicals, investigators have attempted to gauge what acute toxic effects—if any—chemicals may have and to establish what is often described as a safe level of exposure. The goal of this testing, in other words, has been to discover how much of a substance an individual can be exposed to before adverse effects result. Such tests have often entailed conducting experiments designed to determine how much of a given substance would kill a lab animal, usually a mouse, rat, or rabbit.

A look through government databases of chemical safety information, including those compiled in the United States by the Environmental

Protection Agency (EPA) and the Occupational Health and Safety Administration (OSHA), and internationally by the World Health Organization (WHO) and the European Environment Agency, to name but a few, reveals frequent use of the acronym NOEL or NOAEL. These letters stand for "No Observed Effect Level" or "No Observed Adverse Affect Level." As defined by WHO, NOEL or NOAEL is the greatest amount or concentration of a substance found by observation or experiment to cause no detectable effect.

The assumption has been that the greater the measurable amount of exposure—or the greater the dose—the greater the impact. Typically, legally regulated exposure levels have been established based on the NOEL idea of the highest dose that produces no observable effect. These calculations have also generally been based on controlled situations where it's possible to measure the extent of exposure—as in a workplace—rather than the kind of exposure that takes place under more environmentally variable circumstances. Concurrent exposure to multiple contaminants—a common occurrence for most of us—has not been part of these calculations of potential harm. As a result, typical safety standards for hazardous chemical exposure can easily and often fail to fully encompass how most people typically encounter these substances.

The conventional approach to assessing toxicity is also better suited to capturing adverse effects that occur relatively quickly rather than those that may take a long time to become apparent, such as the case with many reproductive and developmental problems (including those resulting from prenatal exposure) or slow-to-manifest diseases like cancer. This approach is also proving far from ideal for identifying substances—like many endocrine-disrupting chemicals—that produce adverse health impacts at very low levels. With these limitations in method, explains John Peterson Myers, chief scientist of the nonprofit organization Environmental Health Sciences, "Toxicology as has been practiced is highly likely to underestimate hazards."[1]

This is the framework on which U.S. laws—and until very recently nearly all such laws—intended to protect environmental and public health from hazardous chemical exposure are based. The Food, Drug, and Cosmetic Act, passed in 1938, was created to set standards for food labeling and requires premarket safety testing for cosmetics, drugs, and medical devices, but until passage of the Toxic Substances Control Act (TSCA) in 1976, there was no national inventory of the chemicals used commercially and no legal requirement for premarket safety testing of such substances. Nor was there any law to restrict or bar sale and use of chemicals with significant adverse health and environmental impacts. And while it may sound as if it does, TSCA as currently configured does relatively little to actually control the majority of chemicals now in commercial production and circulation.

TSCA now serves primarily as an inventory of chemicals manufactured or used commercially in the United States. For what are considered "new" chemicals under the law, TSCA requires chemical manufacturers to submit to the EPA for review a "premanufacture notice," with information about these substances' use, environmental release, and potential human exposure. But TSCA does not cover all the chemicals we encounter by way of consumer products. It leaves review of cosmetics, drugs, food additives, substances used solely as pesticides, and nuclear materials and munitions to other pollution-prevention and product-safety laws. Also excluded from review under TSCA are what the EPA describes as "products of incidental reactions, products of end-use reactions, mixtures (but not mixture components), impurities, byproducts, substances manufactured solely for export, nonisolated intermediates, and substances formed during the manufacture of an article."[2]

These exclusions are important to remember when considering how many synthetic chemicals are active environmentally and biologically, degrading into smaller, more biochemically active (and therefore potentially more hazardous) molecules once in air, water, soil, or inside living organisms. There are also toxic compounds that can be formed when two ingredients in a product created from many react to each other. One such substance—known to be a skin irritant and considered by the EPA to be an "emerging contaminant"—is the compound 1,4 dioxane that can occur when some oxides and ethylene compounds used in many polymers and surfactants (soaps and lotions, for example) are combined.[3] That a

material like PVC will release dioxins when burned, that a commercial
PBDE mixture may carry dioxin traces, or that deca-BDE may break
down into a molecular form of PBDE banned for its toxicity are not covered by TSCA.

Also excluded from this review are "existing" chemicals, the 62,000 or
so that were in production and use when TSCA went into effect in 1979.
They were "grandfathered" into the program without review provisions
and generally assumed to be safe. Of the 80,000 chemicals now listed under TSCA, about 30,000 are in active use and of these about 8,000 are produced at volumes that range from 10,000 to 1 million or more pounds a
year. The United States now has several voluntary programs set up to col-
lect and make available information on various chemicals and their hazards, namely the EPA's High Production Volume Information System and
the Chemical Assessment and Management Program, as well as such industry programs as the American Chemistry Council's Responsible Care
initiative. But overall in the United Sates—and until 2008 in Europe—
measures for eliminating exposure to hazardous chemicals on the job, at
home, and in the environment have been slow, cumbersome, and less
than fully effective.

The European Union's recently implemented REACH (Registration,
Evaluation, and Authorization of Chemicals, effective as of June 1, 2007)
legislation requires manufacturers to prove their products are safe before
they go onto the market—a law that applies to all such substances sold or
used in Europe—and applies to existing as well as new chemicals. Chemicals deemed a significant threat to human health or the environment,
those that are carcinogens, mutagens, or reproductively toxic, will require
special permission to use and then only with specific restrictions. It also
requires that alternatives to the most dangerous be used when such are
available.[4] So in effect, REACH flips the burden from proving harm, as is
the regulatory practice now in the United States, to proving safety.

To be restricted or taken off the market under TSCA, the EPA must
show that the chemical in question presents an unreasonable health or
environmental risk, that human exposure is significant, *and* that existing
information about environmental and health impacts is insufficient to

answer questions about these hazards. Given these hurdles, since 1979, only five chemicals—or categories of chemicals—have been restricted by TSCA: asbestos, chlorofluorocarbons (CFCs), dioxins, hexavalent chromium, and PCBs, although to date even this has not barred the sale of all asbestos products.

As Derek Muir of Environment Canada notes, little attention has been paid to older materials and to substances like polymers (TSCA lists more than 25,000 polymers—compounds that include PVC, polycarbonates, and perfluorinated compounds) because they were not intended to be biologically active and therefore were assumed to be safe. "Between 1985 and about 2005, no one was really looking at the grandfathered-in chemicals," says Muir.[5] And of course TSCA cannot control what's already in the environment—for example, most of the dioxins and PCBs that are currently being detected in people, wildlife, air, soil, and water. Put simply, the net result has thus been more and more people—and the environment—exposed to more and more chemicals.

One practical upshot of the current approach to chemical toxicity and regulatory framework is use of numerous synthetic chemicals long after identification of their environmental and health hazards. Another is a failure to prevent the proliferation of new materials with chemical structures and behaviors comparable to known toxics for which they have been—and are—marketed as alternatives. Brominated flame retardants are one illustration of this problem, but they are far from an isolated case.

This scenario of new materials with comparable intrinsic hazards being offered as alternatives to restricted products is now being repeated with perfluorinated compounds (PFCs). This is a family of compounds with an alphabet soup of names that are used to create nonstick, stain-repellant, and waterproof surfaces and films for both industrial and consumer applications—compounds so widely used that the EPA describes human exposure to these chemicals as "ubiquitous."[6] Perfluorinated compounds also provide an illustration of how difficult it is under our current chemical regulatory system to find out what is in a commercially marketed synthetic chemical even when it's being used in contact with food or in products that touch our bodies. They also demonstrate clearly why

it's so important to ask questions about new materials' biochemical behavior, molecular structure, and behavior—and not simply about performance and expedient production—as they're being designed (rather than
after they're in use) whether they are destined for a pharmaceutical or a
frying pan.

Among this class of synthetic chemicals that we've been wrapping
around food, sitting on, and wearing are substances that have been linked
to impaired liver and thyroid function, immune and reproductive system
problems, altered production of genetic proteins involved in cellular development, to tumor production in lab animals, and to elevated cholesterol
levels in children, as well as to changes in metabolism, including how
the body processes fat. These compounds have endocrine-disrupting-
properties and have been linked to cancer.[7]

These perfluorinated chemicals—also sometimes referred to as perflu-
orocarboxylates (PFCAs) or fluoropolymers—are physically long chain
molecules, made up predominantly of carbons and fluorines, in which
the carbons are surrounded by fluorine atoms. (In chemistry, the prefix
"per" describes a molecule that has the maximum amount of a particular
element for its configuration. In the case of PFCs, each molecule has as
many fluorine atoms attached as that structure can support.) Their varying lengths and structures depend on how, by whom, and for what purpose they are manufactured. This combination of elements makes
strong, flexible, liquid-resistant, and slick-surfaced polymers. They are
used as photoresist compounds in semiconductor manufacture, as fire-
fighting foams, as insulation in plastics that sheathe wires and cables, as
grease-resistant coating on pizza boxes, takeout food containers, microwave popcorn bags, and other packaging, including the support cards
in candy and bakery items. They're also used to make carpets, upholstery,
and clothing fabrics (including leather) stain- and water-resistant—and
are even added to toilet cleaner.

Among these compounds is one known as perfluorooctanoic acid
(PFOA) and another called perfluorooctane sulfonate (PFOS). PFOA—
made with eight carbon atoms and sometimes referred to as C8—is an ingredient of yet another perfluorinated compound called polytetrafluo-

roethylene (PFTE) that made up the original formulation of the products sold under the names Teflon, Gore-Tex, and Scotchguard. The structure that makes PFOA, PFOS, and PFTE so strong and durable also means that they resist degradation in the environment. They do so to such an extent that, like other persistent pollutants, they are chemical globetrotters. They are being found in Arctic animals, both fish and mammals—including polar bears—as well as in ice and snow. They've been found in Lake Ontario trout, in bird eggs collected along the Baltic Sea, in plant tissue, in mink liver, and in threatened and endangered sea turtles along the southern coast of the United States, including the Kemp's Ridley sea turtle, now the scarcest of loggerhead sea turtles. Levels of PFOA and PFOS measured in sea otters along the California coast reported in 2006 were the highest yet found in marine mammals.[8]

While these fluoropolymers and the smaller molecules into which they break down are being found in remote locations and far from where their products were used or made, they are also being detected in human biomonitoring studies all around the world. Testing by the 3M Company—until 2000, itself a major PFOA producer—found PFCs in 95 percent of the Americans it surveyed, while researchers from the Centers for Disease Control found such compounds in 98 percent of the Americans it tested.[9] These compounds have even been found in fetal cord blood of newborn babies. These babies, part of a study conducted in Baltimore, Maryland, were also predominantly low-birth-weight babies, suggesting that there may be a connection between PFC exposure and prenatal development.[10] Subsequent studies found similar incidence of low birth weights in babies born to mothers in Denmark carrying PFOA in their blood.[11] As has been observed in some PBDE studies, PFC levels in children taken from biomonitoring studies appeared to be higher than those for adults in the same studies.[12] Given that PFOA can last for years and that reexposure is almost certain under current conditions, it's not surprising that children have been found to carry proportionally higher loads of these chemicals than do adults.

There are so many of these compounds at large in the environment and PFCs last so long that PFOA has now been detected in deep ocean

environments including in the Labrador Sea, which occupies a critical location in global ocean circulation and could send contaminants into either the European or North American Arctic, thus extending their routes
of potential exposure to people and wildlife.[13] Factor in subsistence and
global warming in the far north and it's likely these contaminants' potential impacts will be felt more directly than in more southerly locations.

Among the factors contributing to the ubiquity of perfluorinated
chemicals is that they have been—and are—being released into the environment from such a variety and so many widely distributed sources, including industrial manufacturing sites. Testing done in the 1980s on behalf of DuPont near its Washington Works facility in Parkersburg, West
Virginia, found high levels of PFOA in the drinking water of nearby communities. In 2002, a similar discovery was made in the municipal and
drinking water sources for over half a dozen Minnesota communities
near the 3M plants that produced the PFCs that went into Scotchguard
and other products. These chemicals were also subsequently found in
both public and private wells and in fish taken from the Mississippi River
and a Minneapolis lake. In late 2008, PFOA and PFOS were found in
sewage sludge used as fertilizer on agricultural fields used for cattle grazing near Decatur, Alabama, where there was fear that the meat itself
might be contaminated. The chemicals are thought to have originated in
wastewater from nearby chemical manufacturing plants.[14] Similar cases
of PFC contamination of waterways and sludge have been reported
across the United States and elsewhere around the world.

Meanwhile, workers at plants that produce PFCs have routinely been
testing positive for these compounds. Such discoveries date back at least
to 1978. Testing of DuPont workers done throughout the 1980s and 1990s
found elevated blood levels of PFOA and employees at DuPont's West
Virginia plant were found—in company studies—also to have higher than
normal rates of leukemia, heart problems, artherosclerosis, and aneu-
rysms. Women at a 3M plant who'd worked with these chemicals reported instances of birth defects in their children in the early 1980s, and in
1997 traces of PFOA and PFOS were reported in donated blood supplies.[15] And as reported by the Centers for Disease control and others,

most people who've been tested carry traces of these chemicals in their blood and urine, whether or not they work with the compounds.

The discovery of PFOA and PFOS contamination from manufacturing plants—and subsequent litigation over 3M's cleanup of the contamination—prompted 3M, the only U.S. producer of PFOS, to discontinue its production of the compound in 2000. The EPA then also restricted the use of PFOS, limiting it to the semiconductor, aviation, and photographic industry processes (these industries can and do import PFOS) but continued to allow domestic production and use of PFOA. Meanwhile, in Europe, accumulating evidence of the persistence and potential health hazards associated with PFOA and PFOS prompted the European Union to pass legislation in 2006 that restricts—but does not entirely ban—use of these compounds, beginning in June 2008.[16]

At about the same time that the EU was formulating its restrictions, the U.S. EPA challenged eight chemical manufacturing companies to voluntarily discontinue PFOA production and eliminate it from their products by 2015. In 2008, the EPA reported that progress had been made toward this goal, with three of the companies reporting 98-percent reduction in U.S. PFOA emissions.[17] The EPA also reports that since the challenge was issued, more than four dozen new alternatives to PFOA have been submitted to the agency for review. Whether this has led to an overall decrease in the use of PFCs is very much open to question. As public concern about exposure to these chemicals has grown, individual states have considered how to take such products out of circulation. California went first, with its state assembly passing a bill in the summer of 2008 that would have barred PFOA from food packaging, but it was vetoed by Governor Arnold Schwarzenegger. Although not an outright ban, perfluorinated compounds are included among those to which alternatives are to be sought under a 2008 New York State "green" procurement act.

While complying with the voluntary EPA program, PFOA producers continued to maintain that their products were safe and posed no risk to human health and—in the case of those contending with cases of local chemical contamination—to resist full acknowledgment of the hazards these chemicals presented. In Minnesota, where 3M PFOA production was linked to adjacent water pollution, under a 2007 agreement, 3M agreed to clean up the source of contamination but not to provide affected communities with alternate drinking water sources until the state of Minnesota could determine safe exposure standards for the perfluorinated compounds in question. Currently there is no firmly established U.S. federal safety standard for PFOA exposure, although a provisional standard for drinking water was set on January 15, 2009. That limit, however, is ten times less stringent, for example, than the current New Jersey state standard.[18]

Despite increasing concern about the environmental and health impacts of pefluorinated compounds and restrictions on PFOA and PFOS, as of May 2007 there were still about fifteen different perfluorinated chemicals used with FDA approval to treat paper and other food packaging. Eight new perfluorinated compounds were approved by the FDA for such uses between 2005 and 2007, some of which were scheduled to go on the market in 2009, according to the Environmental Working Group.[19] Among these substances are coatings for sandwich and burger wrappings, microwave popcorn bags, pizza boxes, French fry wrappings, and muffin papers, making it highly likely that most people will encounter these products at home, in the grocery store, bakery, or a restaurant.

What makes the use of PFCs in these food wrappings of particular concern, note the authors of a 2007 study published in the journal *Environmental Science & Technology*, is that they are being used in contact with greasy and fatty food.[20] The fat, scientists think, provides a vehicle for ingestion of PFCs and allows the long fluoropolymer molecules to break down into smaller, more mobile, and more biologically reactive molecules. These fatty substances are thus thought to be a significant pathway for human exposure to PFCs.

Adding to this concern are documents obtained by *Environmental Science & Technology* under a Freedom of Information Act request revealing that "none of the perfluorinated chemicals currently registered with the FDA has been officially evaluated for its behavior with emulsions or emulsifiers."[21] Among the "emulsions or emulsifiers" with which these food wrapping PFCs might regularly come in contact are substances like butter, margarine or other food oils, fatty foodstuffs like hamburger grease, chocolate icing, and the sauce on a takeout order of Thai noodles. But tracking PFC to such specific exposures is no easy task.[22]

What PFC exposure might mean for people has been highlighted by what Jennifer Keller, a researcher with the Hollings Marine Laboratory in Charleston, South Carolina, and her colleagues have found in their study of endangered loggerhead sea turtles. Keller's team has been measuring levels of PFCs in sea turtles captured along the Carolina coastline, along the Florida coast, and north into the Chesapeake Bay area. Turtles exposed to these chemicals showed signs of liver cell damage and impaired immune systems, conditions that could put them at increased risk for disease.[23] Bottlenose dolphins found in these same locations had even higher levels of PFCs than the turtles studied, probably because dolphins are higher on the food web than sea turtles and thus likely to have greater concentrations of the compounds stored in fat tissue.[24]

"The level of human exposure" to these compounds, says Keller, "is typically comparable or higher to that found in these turtles." Turtles and humans, she explains, have similar immune systems, thus "turtles and people at the current levels of exposure could be suffering the same immune suppression effect." In lab studies these effects have been prompted by very low levels of PFC exposure—levels comparable to what we might routinely now encounter. What this means, Keller suggested, is that what we're exposed to environmentally may no longer be safe.[25]

Still, in 2008, DuPont spokesperson Dan Turner told the *Los Angeles Times*, "Our conclusion is that these products are safe." His company's studies, he said, found no link between high levels of human exposure and the PFCs used in microwave popcorn bags or in packaging used for French fries at fast-food restaurants.[26] DuPont's website in early 2009 continued to maintain confidence in these compounds: "Based on health and toxicological studies, DuPont believes the weight of evidence indicates that PFOA exposure does not pose a health risk to the general public. To date, there are no human health effects known to be caused by PFOA, although study of the chemical continues."[27] Despite its difficulties with the compound, 3M says similarly that "in all of our years of research we have not found any evidence of adverse health effects in our employees."[28]

While new use of PFOA and PFOS may be on the wane, it's not clear that the products being marketed as alternatives are truly environmental improvements. Perhaps even more than the ongoing production of new brominated flame retardants, the current array of PFOA alternatives offers an illustration of how, without asking fundamental questions about molecular design and in the absence of substantial revisions of our current chemical safety assessment and regulatory programs, it's entirely possible that we will continue to eat and cook food that has absorbed synthetic chemicals harmful to human biochemistry.

✢ ✢ ✢

Ever since I first learned about the potential hazards of the chemicals in nonstick coating, I've regarded what had been my favorite rice-cooking pot with sad suspicion. A lovely 2-quart, heavy Dutch oven–type saucepan I'd used happily for years, I've now abandoned it and have been burning rice rather than risk serving up a synthetic chemical that's been shown to give sea turtles tumors. The inside of the pan is scratched and its coating has begun to crumble, and while there is no way I could trace a molecule of that material to anyone's health problems, I just don't feel happy using it. But recently, I walked past an upscale kitchen store in a chic Portland neighborhood that was advertising "environmentally safe" nonstick pans and thought perhaps I could find a replacement for my old pot.

There turn out to be a number of nonstick cookware lines now being sold under the banner of "PFOA-free." Not all are made with the same materials. Upon quick investigation on the website of the company whose ad I'd seen, I discovered that one line of this new cookware being heralded in my eco-friendly town, a product called "Scanpan," actually contains PTFE, the perfluorinated compound that goes into the material trademarked as Teflon. Production of this new coating involves the use of PFOA, so even if very little ends up in each finished product, quantities of PFOA presumably are required to churn out the cookware. There are a number of these PTFE-based "PFOA-free" products now being made by DuPont and other PFC manufacturers.

How, I wondered, could a material be "PFOA-free" yet made with polytetrafluoroethylene (PTFE)? For an explanation, I spoke to Olga Nadeinko, a senior scientist with the Environmental Working Group. These compounds are big, Christmas tree–like polymers, she says, explaining that "the carbon backbone of the molecule is the trunk of the tree and the side chains with the fluorine atoms are the branches." PFOA is also known as C8 because it has eight carbon atoms from which its fluorine branches stem. One of the new perfluorinated compounds being used as an alternative to PFOA or C8, she explains, is a compound known as perfluorohexanoic acid (PFH_xA)—or C6, so named for the six carbon atoms in the molecules that make up the backbone or tree trunk of this PFC.

"What happens," Nadeinko continued, "is that eventually the branches break off the tree" and these branches that form the six-, seven-, and eight-carbon-chain molecules are among the perfluorinated compounds now being found in children and adults. "In the human body, PFOA can last two to fourteen years—on average five—and honestly, you don't want it there," says Nadeinko.[29] And these fluorine branches, she points out, can break off PFC trees with six carbons in their initial formulation just as they can from those with eight carbons.

Yet DuPont, one of the several companies offering products based on C6 chemistry, states that these Capstone products "are based on short chain molecules that cannot break down to PFOA in the environment."[30] The technology used to produce this new product, we're told, requires "negligible PFOA and PFOA precursor content." While the company maintains that these products are not made with PFOA, it also says that it "believes that no one can substantiate statements that fluorotelomer products [the basis of this chemistry] are 'PFOA Free' or have 'Zero PFOA' even if test results are below the limit of detection."[31] This circular statement would seem to indicate that while these products are being marketed as "PFOA-free," they actually may contain—and therefore be made with—these compounds.

That these new products may contain only tiny amounts of PFOA or be made with C6 rather than C8 may not guarantee that they are not perpetuating the environmental or health hazards associated with the older suite of perfluorinated compounds. Scientists are now investigating exactly how and under what circumstances the longer PFCs break down into the shorter, more biologically active molecules. Studies thus far suggest that these active compounds may be entering the environment from all commercially marketed fluorinated polymers.[32] Toxic effects observed have resulted not only from C8 but also from exposure to C6, and it appears that very small amounts—in micromolar concentrations—can produce adverse effects.

Such low-level effects again point to the difficulty in relying on a chemical regulatory system based on toxicology oriented toward the effects of high-dose exposures. "The chemical industry is doing a pretty good job right now at preventing people from dying on the shop floor. This was not so a hundred years ago," comments Terry Collins, professor of chemistry at Carnegie Mellon University and director of Carnegie Mellon's Institute for Green Science.[33] We've become practiced at identifying acute toxicological endpoints, says Collins—who, along with John Warner and Paul Anastas, is one of the leading green chemistry advocates—"chemicals that kill and chemicals that interact with DNA, causing mutations that lead to cancer." But the discovery of endocrine-disrupting chemicals, of "chemicals that interact with cellular development," and may do so at low doses, he explains, caused "a tectonic plate shift" in where we need to look for health hazards and how we think about toxicity.

"The underlying assumption that the chemical industry has been built on," Collins continues, "assumes that any useful chemical commercialized for anything other than drug purposes will not have a profound impact on human health and the environment. Our most common chemical screens are designed to identify chemicals that kill," not chemicals that interfere with finely tuned hormonal feedback loops—as has turned out to be the case with PFOA and other perfluorinated compounds that have endocrine-disrupting effects.

Over the past ten years or so, increasingly sophisticated research techniques have begun to pinpoint the mechanisms of the subtle but potentially extensive effects of endocrine-disrupting compounds. A pattern has emerged in that results of exposure to some of these chemicals are often far from linear—and in some cases, high doses of a chemical can not only produce no effect but may even prompt the opposite effect from what a low dose causes, as appears to be the case with bisphenol A. Scientists can now locate the precise genetic receptors where many such chemical interactions occur and have learned that certain synthetic chemicals have molecular compositions and structures that enable them to interact with the site where a hormone would bind. This has been discovered for a number of common synthetic chemicals, including bisphenol A and the other chemicals Bruce Blumberg of UC Irvine called "obesogens," for dioxins, and for perfluorinated compounds.

If one of these interloper or xenobiotic chemicals occupies one of these gene sites, it can trigger an alternate sequence of events that can upset an organism's healthy balance and lead to disease. I came to picture this as a kind of Rube Goldberg machine with events set in motion not by falling buckets and leaping cats, but by chemicals and genetic material that operate on a cellular and molecular scale. What appears to happen in some circumstances is that a very small amount of one of these biologically alien compounds can prompt this chain of events, while a large amount may "flood" or overwhelm the binding site (the genetic receptor) and actually shut down any possible reaction. And sometimes, as Frederick vom Saal has seen in bisphenol A's trigger of fat-cell production, such flooding or overload can set in motion a completely different biochemical response than would a minute amount of chemical prompt.

Timing is also a key factor in determining what sort of response to endocrine effecting chemicals will prompt. "You need to look at all life stages," Ted Schettler tells me. What happens at one point in life may not happen at another even with precisely the same exposure. These are among the chemical contamination hazards that can be swept under the rug when safety assurances—and regulatory standards—are based on promises that exposure may be to only trace quantities of biologically active compounds.

Another feature of our current chemical regulatory system that has effectively perpetuated the potential for continued exposure to hazardous materials is that the Toxic Substances Control Act allows manufacturers to claim confidentiality and withhold full details of a material's composition. This is one of the great problems with products like the new perfluorinated compounds being marketed as safer alternatives to existing problematic materials. That this information is proprietary makes it extremely difficult for consumers or scientists to make independent assessments of the products. For example, the twenty-three Material Safety Data Sheets (MSDS) for perfluorinated Capstone products available through DuPont's website include many for which no exposure limits have been set, and materials with general or obscure descriptions such as "fluorinated acrylic polymer," "NJ Trade Secret Registry #00850201001-5738P," and "Proprietary Surfactant Package," as well as many compounds with no Chemical Abstracts Service (CAS) number—the number assigned by the American Chemical Society to every chemical compound that's been described in the scientific literature. Adding to the obscurity, a number of these data sheets describe the exposure effects of ingredients other than the fluorinated material and none caused by the perfluorinated compound itself.[34]

A search for toxicity information on one Capstone product ingredient listed on an MSDS sheet led me to a database maintained by the U.S. EPA's Office of Pollution Prevention and Toxics. There, under a confidential CAS number and confidential submitter of toxicity testing, were the results of tests assessing whether or not the substance, polyfluorosulfonic acid, causes chromosomal aberrations in hamster ovary cells. The downloadable public copy of the tests results filed on October 30, 2007, is labeled "Company Sanitized" and thus had nothing to identify who conducted the tests or manufactures the material. Test results showed "substantial cytotoxicity" (50 percent inhibition of normal cell growth was observed) as well as "statistically" and "biologically significant" evidence that exposure caused chromosomal abnormalities. The filing of unpublished information about new chemicals satisfies current EPA reporting requirements for producers, distributors, and importers of compounds even when such data "may lead to a conclusion of substantial risk to human health or the environment."[35] Clearly, transparency is not a feature of this system of compiling and disseminating information.

This, however, was not the only obscurity one might encounter in a search for information about "PFOA-free" nonstick pans. As I investigated further, I learned from the Scanpan website that while some of these pans seem to contain PFTE (the PFOA-containing compound), the company is also launching a new "PFOA-free" coating for these pans called "Green-Tek." Scanpan and other companies describe such lines of "PFOA-free," nonstick cookware as "hard anodized" surfaces with "patented ceramic-titanium technology." One company describes a surface created from sand, "one of nature's most abundant and renewable resources," but none offer anything approaching detailed material information.

Unable to track down specifics of materials used in these pots and pans (brand names include GreenTek by Scanpan, Circulon, and Earth-Pan), I did a bit of sleuthing to find out something about other widely available lines of "PFOA-free" pans sold under different brand names, including GreenPan. These GreenPan lines of cookware, I learned from the company's website, are rendered nonstick with something called Thermalon, a trademarked product made by a company of the same name based in Busan, South Korea, and in Hong Kong.

According to its manufacturer, Thermalon uses what the company calls a "polymer ceramic nano-composite for the nonstick coating."[36] A simplified chemical equation on the company's website—which devotes much of its space to explaining the hazards of PTFE but offers much less information about the company or what the product actually contains—indicates the material to be a polymer made of silicon, carbon, hydrogen, and oxygen. No other information on the material's composition is available. According to its manufacturer, however, Thermalon does not leach lead, chromium, arsenic, cadmium, or antimony—none of which you'd want mixed into your supper. Nor does the Thermalon coating dissolve or otherwise leach into solutions of sulfuric acid, sodium hydroxide (also known as lye), xylene, or methyl ethyl ketone—none of which one would expect the home dishwasher to encounter. Thermalon also apparently complies with the U.S. Food and Drug Administration requirements for indirect food additives.

Digging further, I also learned that in January 2008 the Shin Woo Trading Company, the South Korean company that had been manufacturing the coating materials for these nonstick "GreenPans," merged with Thermalon, the company that markets the product, which described itself as the "fastest growing company in the environmentally friendly coating industry for 2007." The announcement of the merger with Shin Woo, which received wide coverage in business news bulletins, noted a forthcoming investment of $15 million. When I searched this information late in the summer of 2008, the Home Shopping Network was selling the pans, Martha Stewart had a line as did Cuisinart and the British manufacturer Russell Hobbs, known for its high-end electric tea kettles. Retail advertising claims these pans have reportedly earned a literal Good Housekeeping Seal of Approval.[37] But what is this material actually made of?

According to one website aimed at a Japanese and international Asian market, the Shin Woo Trading company describes its core business as an "importer, distributor, and manufacturer of phenol injection resin from China. Now expending [sic] export business to China and other countries with nonstick ceramic coating agents."[38] I also uncovered the description of a patent filed in May 2007 by Shin Woo Trading Company, Ltd., for a nonstick coating for aluminum-based cookware. The coating is apparently a layered material involving a ceramic coating made with silicon oxide and a filler that may include any one or more of a dozen or so minerals, manufactured in a process that involves the use of nano-sized titanium dioxide (a material now under scrutiny for potential adverse environmental and health effects) and two industrial chemicals for which there is very little if any literature on ecological or health impacts.[39] The minerals listed on the publicly available patent information include barium, cesium, strontium, and several substances rendered in transliterated Korean. Is this material safe? From the information available, it's not possible to tell.

What all this says is that we continue to create new synthetic materials, some based on compounds known to be persistent and hazardous, others based on brand-new compounds and technologies with unknown health and environmental impacts, and allow them to be launched into high-volume production and used in widely distributed consumer products—some intended for use with food and on our bodies—without any independent testing of their biological safety. In the United States we—and that includes government agencies—continue to rely on manufacturers to assure of us their products' safety in a system that, despite voluminous databases and electronically filed documents, has little real transparency.

What's been happening with perfluorinated chemicals, particularly the marketing of the C6 products based on chemistry comparable to a known toxic (C8) as "green," speaks to the urgent need for a way to protect against the view that simply labeling a product "green" somehow makes it so. At the same time, this story also provides a clear example of how relying on a list of barred materials to protect environmental and public health offers little real assurance of safety. This underscores what green chemistry guru Paul Anastas calls the "importance of recognizing the molecular basis of toxicity and regulating it"—as opposed to continuing our historical approach of regulating by minimizing exposure.[40] Combine these issues of labeling and transparency with the problems posed by continuing to rely on a regulatory framework based on what is arguably now outdated toxicology and risk assessment, and it seems clear that there is an urgent need not only for materials redesign but also for an overhaul of the policies that determine chemical safety.

CHAPTER EIGHT

Nanotechnology

Perils and Promise of the Infinitesimal

What do a pair of Dockers brand "Go" khaki pants, a Wilson tennis racket, Burt's Bees "Chemical Free" sunscreen, a Samsung washing machine, Land's End earmuffs, a face cream from fashion house Chanel, and my Apple laptop computer have in common with a billion-dollar U.S. government program, a Berkeley, California, city ordinance, and a novel about invisible robots run amok?[1] All involve what are called nanomaterials, synthetic materials engineered at the microscopic scale of one to 100 nanometers—a nanometer being *one-billionth* of a meter. To get a sense of the scale it helps to know that a human hair is about *80,000* nanometers wide. This is so small it can mean manipulating materials at the atomic level.[2]

What makes nanomaterials so unlike the materials with which we are more familiar—and is the source of both their promise and their potential perils—is that at this infinitesimal scale materials change in fundamental ways. Not only are nanomaterials so small that they may be able to penetrate skin and cell membranes and so get to places that their conventionally sized counterparts cannot, but as Vicki Colvin, professor of chemistry and director of the Center for Biological and Environmental Nanotechnology at Rice University, explains, "Size changes chemistry."[3]

143

At the nano-scale, materials have surface areas and geometries that give them chemical, physical, and biological properties that may be completely different than those they possess at the macro or even micro scale. They can take on new optical properties that allow them to absorb special wavelengths of light, lending themselves to applications like dyes and medical tracers. Elements like gold, aluminum, or carbon, for example, which are without inherent biological activity at conventional sizes, can interact in ways that would not otherwise be expected when engineered into nanomaterials. These reactions can—again, for example—be directed toward creating polymers, developing materials that detoxify pollutants, and constructing those that will knit wounded cell membranes. It is precisely these novel characteristics and possibilities that make nanomaterials such intriguing chemical tools. These properties are also what enable them to behave in ways that we do not yet fully understand and that are prompting widespread concern about their environmental and health impacts.

These concerns have given rise to science fiction scenarios of runaway molecules replicating and invading—Michael Crichton's "nanobots" and Eric Drexler's "gray goo"—but also to a serious public discourse that has the potential to bring about a sea change in how we consider new materials and technologies. And while there is nothing intrinsically "green" about nanotechnology per se (it can use toxic elements and produce hazardous materials just as conventionally sized synthetic chemistry can), it is this new universe of chemical behaviors—particularly the potential to create more resource-efficient materials—along with the opportunity to establish a more proactive approach to the safety of new materials than currently exists, that presents important opportunities for green chemistry.

On the performance side, at the nano-scale, novel reactions made possible at this size can in some instances eliminate the need for reagents (process chemicals used to induce other chemical reactions) that can be hazardous and expensive, and thus both environmentally and economically costly. This reactivity can also be used to make molecules bind effectively and efficiently in ways that can create layered surfaces and polymers and repair damaged materials. It can also be put to work detoxifying or otherwise destroying unwanted molecules without the use of additional chemicals, giving nanomaterials great potential in the realm of stain removal and chemical remediation. All these are applications that, if accomplished without hazard, meet green chemistry goals.

But unusual properties also require new ways of assessing these new materials' potential toxicity, environmental disruption, and health hazards. Existing test methods simply do not encompass all the possible ways in which nanomaterials can interact. Nanomaterials behave so differently from other materials that even cleaning a spill means stopping to think whether or not one can safely reach for a vacuum cleaner or a mop. And standard personal protection equipment may not be what's required to ensure safety for those working with nanomaterials in a lab or manufacturing plant.

These many unknowns are also prompting leading nanotechnology practitioners to call for ways of investigating nanomaterials' environmental and health impacts—and disseminating this information—that are substantially different than those that have been used historically. Yet despite these cautions, nanomaterials have been proliferating so quickly that in early 2009 researchers estimated that it could cost U.S. industries over a billion dollars and take more than fifty years to conduct toxicity testing for the various nanomaterials already in existence.[4]

While nanomaterials are turning up in items as mundane as hats and underwear, the scientists who work with them are exploring a terrain that is in its way as exotic as the deep ocean or outer space. Some nanomaterial names even sound exotic: quantum dots, carbon nanotubes, fullerenes. Nanomaterials can only be viewed under high-powered microscopes, but even a quick glimpse through such a lens offers a clear picture of how materials change at this scale. For instead of seeing the seamless flat surface of a solid snip of metal, for example, what you see is something resembling a honeycomb or grate or a series of slices of a sphere or in the case of nanoparticles of carbon, something that resembles multiple strands of hair or thread. It is this expanded, multidimensional molecular territory with which scientists are working—both physically and chemically—as they manipulate nanoparticles.

It is by exploiting the scale-dependent properties—which, depending on the material, enable nanomaterials to reflect or absorb certain wavelengths of light, bind with, and destroy undesirable bacteria or tumor cells—that nanomaterials are being put to work in products that range from improved cancer treatment, more efficient solar cells, faster computers, and cleaner water to stain-resistant neckties, smell-resistant socks, and toothpaste that promises whiter teeth. Nanomaterials are being used as antibacterial agents, catalysts that remediate pollution, and as drug-delivery vehicles. They can also create incredibly strong and light building materials (this is why nanomaterials are attractive for aircraft and sports gear) and can be used to create semiconductor circuitry. An inventory compiled by the Woodrow Wilson Center's Project on Emerging Nano-technologies—the only such comprehensive compilation to date of nanomaterial-infused products—lists more than 800 consumer products containing nanomaterials, a list that does not include specialized medical or industrial applications.[5]

Among the behaviors that distinguish nanomaterials—and why they are attracting green chemists—is how they lend themselves to applications that can be used to reduce waste within the manufacturing process. Take the fact that these tiny particles can be engineered and combined in ways that eliminate the need for additional process chemicals and other potentially costly resources to spur a chemical reaction. This is often described by those in the field as a "bottom-up" approach to chemical synthesis or, to use a phrase that has helped spur fears of "nanobots," "self-assembly." What this means is working with the molecules' existing nature, putting them in a position of natural attractions and reactions rather than pushing them into reactions that require applied force, whether chemical or physical. (Hence the self-assembly and possibility for replication.) Reducing or doing away with the need for solvents and additional steps in a chemical synthesis or manufacture of chemical-intensive products like semiconductors and pharmaceuticals has great potential in terms of reducing overall resource use and the potential for harmful byproducts, environmental impacts, and health hazards. But to ensure that substituting one set of materials for another doesn't simply create new hazards, big and hard questions need to be asked about nanomaterials.

These materials and their properties are so new that Barbara Karn of the EPA's Office of Research and Development calls the advent of nanotechnology a paradigm shift. "In science we assume that no matter how much we slice a material, its properties are retained. At nano-scale, this is not the case and it's counterintuitive to the way we've been working," she told me.[6]

"Size-dependent properties are what make nanomaterials powerful," explains James Hutchinson, professor of organic and materials chemistry and director of the Materials Science Institute at the University of Oregon.[7] Size is also the primary cause for concern about nanomaterials' implications for human health and the environment, as Vicki Colvin explains: It's nanoparticles' large surface areas that open the possibility for biological interactions. This means that a material that is environmentally benign when used at a larger scale—such as the conventionally sized titanium dioxide used as a masking agent in sunscreen—has the potential to behave completely differently when used as nanoparticles.

While the skin may be an effective barrier against a substance at the micro scale, for example, nanoparticles of the same material may be able to permeate skin and other cellular membranes. These minute particles may be able to enter the bloodstream, to permeate lung tissue, or to target specific organs, including the brain. With specially designed medical or pharmaceutical products, this may be desirable and even highly beneficial. But nanomaterials that reach organs unintentionally present the possibility for adverse impacts. "We don't yet have a good grasp of how nanoparticles change in the human body," says Kristen Kulinowski, director of the International Council of Nanotechnology (ICON).[8] She and her colleagues at Rice University in Texas are working to develop models that will assess the behavior of nanomaterials in biological settings, something about which relatively little is known.

So what does happen when we are exposed to products containing nanomaterials? How does the exposure to nanoparticles one may get by applying a nano-sunscreen, wearing socks with an antimicrobial nanomaterial, or using a golf club made with a nano-carbon affect health? Or do they affect health at all? What about exposure to nanomaterials for people working in factories or laboratories where these products are made? What happens when these products are disposed of? Right now, these questions about the potential hazards of nanomaterials are just beginning to be answered, and one of the challenges is that assessing these materials adds considerable complexity to considerations of biological activity and toxicity.

Risk changes significantly when you make a transition to the use of materials at the nano-scale, Colvin points out. "Any new technology brings new risks," she says, citing the examples of DDT that helped curb malaria, pesticides that improved crop yields yet turned out to be human carcinogens, and efficient refrigerants that led to the ozone hole. Clearly one of the looming questions is: Can we do better job of dealing with these hazards and risks than we have in the past?

But, cautions Colvin's colleague Kristen Kulinowski, "we don't want to throw the baby out with the bathwater. The medical applications have enormous promise. There could indeed be a cure for cancer. There's enormous promise for bioremediation products. The goal is not to condemn or exonerate nanotechnology because we don't yet have answers about product behavior, but to head off or anticipate problems before they occur—not just in post-market scrutiny"—that is, after they are already in the marketplace.

What makes this even more complicated is that in addition to their novel size-dependent properties, nanomaterials are also structurally complex. James Hutchinson of OSU explains that nanomaterials are typically engineered to have what's called a core and a coating—a shell made out of one material surrounding a core of another. Both core and shell can vary in size (or thickness) and chemical composition. These variations will determine how a nanomaterial interacts with other substances, and thereby influence a nanomaterial's biological activity and, hence, potential toxicity. Those working in nanotechnology call this set of variations on a set of chemical combinations a "library" of materials.

As this is being explained to me, I remember exercises from my elementary school "new math" workbooks where we were asked to list permutations based on a list of ingredients: how many different combinations could you make, we were asked, given a hot dog, ketchup, mustard, sauerkraut, cheese, lettuce, mayonnaise, and two slices of bread. Add a hamburger to this list, and see how the variations expand. Now imagine that the behavior of that hamburger or hot dog—the taste, the smell, how it could be digested, and even its nutrients—might completely change depending on the addition of condiments and you begin to get an idea of what's involved in assessing libraries of nanomaterials. "Nanomaterials have dynamically changing surfaces, kind of like the corona of the sun," explains Kulinowski. So to understand a nanomaterial's environmental impacts, one must assess the behavior of a whole suite of these variations.

Part of the research going on at Colvin's lab at Rice and Hutchinson's at the University of Oregon is a systematic attempt to characterize "libraries" of nanomaterials in order to understand their environmental impacts. This will help develop what Hutchinson calls "design rules"—or guidelines—intended to prevent creation of hazardous and toxic products. "Will there be any really nasty surprises coming from nano?" asks Terry Collins, director of the Institute for Green Oxidation Chemistry at Carnegie Mellon University. "People in chemistry get excited by technical performance. But we can't assume there will be no interactions with humans and we need to be aware that at the molecular scale of nanomaterials, barriers present for larger materials will not be present. At the molecular scale, these substances can permeate our bodies relatively easily. There are an unbelievable number of interactions that are possible," he says, "so we need to be very careful."

These unknowns have prompted calls for caution from government agencies, academics, and citizen groups—in May and June of 2007 alone more than half a dozen such reports were released—and have since been followed by many more.[9] A number of scientists working in the field, however, including Colvin, Collins, Hutchinson, and Karn see this concern as an opportunity to ask questions vital to protecting human health and the environment from what have often been called the "unintended consequences" of new materials and technologies. Their interest led in 2008 to the creation of the International Alliance for NanoEHS (Environmental Health and Safety) Harmonization, organized by a group of materials scientists and toxicologists from the United States, Europe, and Japan who will work on developing environmental, health, and safety standards for nanomaterials, standards that do not currently exist.[10] This information will be available to scientists worldwide, and funding for this work will come from the participants' research institutions rather than from sponsors of a particular material or product. Both the extent of information-sharing planned and the noncommercial funding represent a departure from the traditional approach to both commercial chemistry and evaluation of its products.

"We need to learn from the past and think about issues of safety and sustainability as early as possible," says Colvin. "We need to engineer materials as safe materials from the beginning to understand the mechanisms of toxicity," she says, so they can be incorporated into the design and application of new materials. Given the chemistry and geometry of nanomaterials, understanding the full behavior of these molecules, whether they're destined for consumer products, pharmaceuticals, or industrial applications, requires even more scrutiny than it does with conventionally sized materials.

In advocating for this design-stage approach to new material safety, what Colvin, Collins, Hutchinson, and their colleagues are aiming to foster is a merging of green chemistry with nano-science. Hutchinson has called this a "proactive approach" to nanotechnology, with a goal of creating new materials with "high performance that pose minimal harm to human health and the environment."[11]

"Some of the same questions to ask about nano are the same questions we should be asking about any chemical materials," says Paul Anastas, director of the Center for Green Chemistry and Green Engineering at Yale University. "Can the substance get into the body? Can it be inhaled or absorbed into the skin? What does the substance do to the body and what does the body do to the substance? Is it persistent or bioaccumulative? Does it contain known toxics?" Anastas also cites the need for life-cycle analyses of nanomaterial to ensure that those that are deemed safe will be produced sustainably—to make sure the environmental footprint of the entire production process does not undermine the apparent efficiencies of using nanotechnology. But thus far, says Anastas, "these questions are only being asked by a fraction of practitioners."[12]

"Just like the rest of chemistry, nanotechnology is not exempt from biology," Collins points out. For example, "we need to understand that it's not a good idea to make a distributive technology [a product that's going to be produced at high volume and widely distributed] with a known hazardous substance such as cadmium. If you don't stay away from toxic elements, nanotechnology is just another way of distributing toxics."[13]

The complexity and many variations on the use of particular elements in nanomaterials makes assessing their toxicity a challenge that's been compounded thus far by a lack of clarity and agreement about what results of such testing actually mean. Right now, particularly where consumer products are concerned (where nanomaterials are inconsistently labeled at best), the kind of nanomaterials being used and any safety information that might exist for them are generally unknown. Given our experience thus far with unexplained new substances, erring on the side of caution is an easy impulse to understand. Nanomaterials also raise the issue of appropriate technology. If, for example, conventional materials work perfectly well in a lip balm, why introduce elements of the unknown by using a nanomaterials-infused product instead?

Colvin, only partially jesting, calls discussion of dangerous nanoparticles the "Darth Vader" side of nanotechnology. This dark side includes accidentally or incidentally produced nanomaterials that may unintentionally be inhaled or absorbed through the skin—and speculation about the impacts. Recently published papers indicate that inhaled nanoparticles of titanium dioxide and iron oxide may cause adverse impacts to lung tissue cells and that single-walled carbon nanotubes may cause damage to cardiovascular tissue and cause damage to lung tissue like that caused by asbestos fibers, for example.[14] There is also some evidence that nanoparticles of titanium dioxide, such as those that are already in many sunscreens, as well as nanoparticles of other metals—zinc, copper, and silver—can damage beneficial bacteria, an impact that has the potential to harm soil and aquatic ecosystems.[15]

Part of the difficulty in assessing nanomaterials' safety and behavior is that we don't yet have templates in place to guide us to the appropriate questions. The current standard Material Safety Data Sheet poses questions about a material's behavior, which many environmental safety experts and advocates consider far from adequately rigorous for any materials, treats nanomaterials simply like macro or bulk materials. Yet already, workers are shaping materials based on nano-scale carbon, for example, into elements of aircraft, specialized technical machinery, and more ordinary things like bicycle frames. So it is crucial to know what sort of respirator, protective mask, or other gear will effectively block these infinitesimally small particles from reaching nose, eyes, mouth, and skin. Understanding nanomaterials' behavior is key to understanding what sort of personal protective equipment might be needed. Again, nanomaterials' size-dependent properties adds to the challenge.

As an example of nanomaterials' complexity, Colvin explains that evidence thus far indicates that some nanomaterials constructed from carbon are environmentally benign, while others, in aggregated form, can be very toxic. Scientists working with nanomaterials however, are also quick to point out that nanoparticles do occur naturally and their properties have been used throughout history. But isolating these particles, creating engineered nanomaterials, and putting them into high-volume commercial production and into widely distributed consumer products is very different from knowing that it's the optical properties of nanoparticles of metal that impart color to stained glass.

To illustrate how many variations of a single substance used at nanoscale can complicate issues of toxicity, Colvin gives the example of a carbon nanostructure known as Carbon-sixty or C_{60}. In some configurations, C_{60} is extremely hydrophobic and tends to gravitate toward oils and fats or lipids, and under certain circumstance will destroy fats in cell membranes and thus be very cytotoxic—poisonous to cells in general. But in other configurations, C$_{60}$—the discovery of which won a Nobel Prize—is now being used to create specifically targeted drugs and to build artificial membranes.

Even more difficult to assess than how nanomaterials will behave in a controlled or constricted environment—including within a cell—is how they will behave when released to the global environment. While some studies have shown certain nanomaterials to have little impact on soil microbes (to offer one example of environmental behavior) some nanomaterials have been engineered specifically to destroy microbes, while others not intended to damage bacteria apparently do.[16] Andrew Maynard, science adviser to the Woodrow Wilson Center Project on Emerging Nanotechnologies, poses a question about antimicrobial nanomaterials similar to one that has been running through my head. What we're talking about are the nanoparticles of silver that are now being used to keep socks and underwear odor-free. "They're reasonably safe under certain circumstances," says Maynard. "But in the environment, what would happen over time?" he asks. What would happen after disposal of the finished product that contains these nanomaterials or the disposal of the antimicrobial agent itself? "Could they carry on killing microbes for years and years, knocking out a bottom layer of the ecosystem?" asks Maynard. At this point we simply don't know.

Dr. Peter Lichty, occupational medical director at the Lawrence Berkeley Laboratory points out that from a laboratory perspective nanomaterials are not dramatically different from other new materials created in the lab. "We create very small quantities of material and follow OSHA lab safety standards and have chemical hygiene plans that protect individuals from materials of unknown properties," he tells me. When the lab disposes of nanomaterials that it has used or created, they're treated as hazardous waste. Lichty also points out that laboratory and commercial production procedures tend to vary significantly. Commercially, speed is often a priority and materials are used in large quantities compared to laboratory use, which is typically more controlled and entails only small quantities that are more easily contained. (This, I think, as he describes commercial production, is where we begin to get into trouble.)

But overall, says, Lichty, despite careful work and precautions, "Toxicity information is not sufficient at this point."[17]

This information gap is what led the Berkeley City Council to initiate conversations with the Lawrence Lab and the University of California that resulted in guidelines for the local production and disposal of nano-materials—the first such ordinance in the United States. Cambridge, Massachusetts—another research hot spot—is now considering community oversight procedures for nanotechnology, and other such regulations are likely to follow elsewhere. "Why did the city do this?" Berkeley city councilor Gordon Wozniak asks rhetorically. "We have a very active citizenry and we're concerned about a lot of things, including health risks in general. There was a general concern that [nanotechnology] was all unknown and we should be careful," he says.[18]

So, Colvin asks, "How do you create a safe system for these materials? How do you make decisions with a science in progress?" Part of what makes developing safety protocols, let alone standards for nanomaterials so complex, Colvin reminds me, is that "there are so many permutations of a nanoparticle that it upends the traditional strategy of single-item toxicology."[19] This means that new safety procedures are needed for handling, working with, and producing nanomaterials—something being called for by industry and scientists, and also now by governments. In 2005, however, less than 4 percent of the U.S. federal spending budget dedicated to nanotechnology was designated for environmental, health, and safety research.[20] In 2007, I was told off-the-record by an EPA official that much of the oversight of nanotechnology that had been done was being carried out not by the federal government but by the Wilson Center and other institutions, although much of this research did receive EPA funding. The implication was that the federal government had fallen behind on the job and that the Bush administration let that happen.

Since then, there has been a litany of reports—including from the National Research Council—pointing out lack of oversight in nanotechnology, the lack of resources currently available for such work within the U.S. Food and Drug Administration and Consumer Product Safety Commission, and the lack of adequate safety testing for nanomaterials currently in consumer products, now processed foods among them. According to the Wilson Center, as of December 2008, the worldwide nanotechnology food market was estimated to grow to more than $20 billion by 2010. By the center's count there were already some 84 consumer products in the food-and-beverage sector that manufacturers claim are nanotechnology products.[21]

There has now also been a flurry of efforts to regulate nanotechnology. In January 2009, a nanotechnology research bill that would increase funding for environmental health and safety work was introduced by Representative Barton Gordon of Tennessee along with twenty-one cosponsors and support from the House Science and Technology Committee. At about the same time, Canada proposed legislation that would require companies using nanotechnology products to detail their use. And under a law passed by the European Union in March 2009 that will become effective in 2012, all cosmetics made with nanomaterials will have to undergo safety testing and have all such ingredients listed if they're to be sold in the EU.[22] But as of April 1, 2009, the United States has no specific provisions for testing the safety of products containing nanomaterials or any labeling requirements for such products.

Currently, for practical purposes—as far as consumer products are concerned—nanomaterials are generally being treated like any other new synthetics that come onto the market. They have been launched into commercial production with little real knowledge of what their long-term environmental or health impacts may be. And while green chemistry advocates like Anastas, Colvin, Collins, and Hutchinson have articulated quite clearly—both in terms of policy and their own work—how important it is to consider the full range of nanomaterials' impacts at the design stage, the products of such thinking have yet to become the norm.

At a "Safer Nano" conference I attended in 2007, I listened to a presentation that described a series of nanomaterials that were layered compounds with reactive properties that can be used in insulation and cooling materials. (One possible application is in vehicle upholstery.) One of the compounds described contained antimony, lead, silver, and tellurium. "Lead. What is lead doing in a 'safer' material?" I wondered. Aren't we now keeping children off playing fields coated with artificial turf because it contains lead dust and taking toys off shelves because of lead contamination? And these now-barred products have big—not nano-scale—particles of lead. After decades of being misled that the lead content in paint was not a health hazard, why should the public accept the assurance that lead in a nanomaterial that heats car seats is not a problem? The amounts of lead in such a product might be so small as to be insignificant even by the most sensitive measures of health effects. On the other hand, the particles might be so small as to create new problems. Again, at this point we just don't know. And the challenge is to figure out how to develop transparent and effective testing that will protect public and environmental health but not impede innovative technology.

Thousands of synthetic chemicals have gone into high production volume and into innumerable consumer products over the past 100 years. Many have later been found to be toxic to human health and the environment. In most cases—with the possible exception of genetically modified and irradiated food—there has been little, if any, public outcry about these substances or technologies prior to the discovery of serious problems. Nanotechnology, with its futuristic-sounding nanotubes and fullerenes, its promise of materials that can self-assemble, and its alluring applications, has captured public attention in an entirely different way. Still, a poll released in December 2008 found that nearly half of the thousand Americans surveyed said they had heard nothing about nanotechnology—an indication that relying on public pressure to result in public health protection may not be adequate.[23]

Precisely because nanomaterials are distinctly different from others, they create a special imperative, says Paul Anastas, "to get things right at the design stage." With nanomaterials, says Anastas, we need to have "innovation by design and not by accident." And because the products are already on store shelves, in our kitchen and bathroom cabinets, it is especially imperative that we begin to catch up with this avalanche of new materials. Anastas adds: "We're on the verge of having a very scared public—irrationally in some cases—if we don't ask the questions that could cut the risks."

If the unknowns of nanotechnology prompt such questions about the environmental and health impacts of these new materials' molecular design—and time is taken to answer them thoroughly *as* these materials are being designed, not *after* they're in commercial use—then, as Terry Collins suggests, "Nano may be bringing green chemistry to the forefront." Clearly, there is a lot of catch-up to do and it will not be easy, but if, as has been proposed, nanotechnology practitioners and innovators collaborate and share information, it might indeed be possible to begin to get this right.

CHAPTER NINE

Material Consequences
Toward a Greening of Chemistry

"I'm a very skeptical scientist," says Terry Collins of Carnegie Mellon's Institute for Green Science. "The stakes of the chemical enterprise are incredibly high." Proponents of green chemistry, I had quickly discovered, are very much on a mission. All speak with an urgency more typical of political and social campaigns than the practice of science. Then I began to realize that, right now, green chemistry entails all three.

"Civilization is highly chemical in its nature," says Collins, a tall, impressively outspoken native of New Zealand. After the invention and commercialization of the first chemical dye in England in the 1850s, he explains, the chemical industry was "off to the races." When he talks about chemistry, Collins likes to put current chemical production in historical context, sometimes taking the story all the way back to the Romans' use of lead.

"If it was 1500 and we were in an Italian hill town, you could only impact the people who you meet. Now every time you turn on the car, you're affecting thousands of children. We can now impact people we never meet with these chemicals. We can affect babies yet to be born. Technology and science have given rise to a whole new category of ethics. There's no precedent for it."

We must eliminate elements such as lead (in batteries) and mercury (in fluorescent lights), and do better with nanotechnology, he tells me. "We need to use only elements that we [ourselves] are made of in catalysts and polymers we're going to make commercially," Collins argues. And it would be better for our health and the environment to use more "recently dead plants rather than fossilized plants—that is, petroleum."

"The underlying assumption that the chemical industry has been built on assumed that any useful chemical commercialized for anything other than drug purposes will not have a profound impact on human health and the environment," suggests Collins, reminding me, just as John Warner and Paul Anastas have, that chemists typically are given no training in toxicology, an oversight Collins likens to "giving people keys to the car with no drivers' training." He also reminds me that of the approximately 80,000 chemicals currently in commerce, only about 4,500 are pharmaceuticals. This means that the vast majority of synthetic chemicals that go into products that surround us were designed with the assumption that their chemical constituents would not be entering our bodies or otherwise affecting ecological systems. "It stretches comprehension and it's a very flawed concept," says Collins, "to think that commercialized chemicals like pesticides will not do anything to us."

"Green chemistry," says Collins, "is a major paradigm shift. And there is no option but for us to do this." But, he points out, "It's easier to say what green chemistry isn't rather than what it is."

"The fundamental concept of green chemistry," Collins tells me, can be spelled out in an equation: "Risk equals exposure times hazard [Risk = Hazard × Exposure]. As green chemists, let's try to understand the hazard and try to get the hazard out. We have to turn the aircraft carrier around and get the hazard out." Another aspect of this metaphorical ship is that we've relied on our preferred energy source—petroleum—to supply the base for so many of our current synthetics. "If you don't have the energy problem fixed, it overwhelms everything else," notes Collins.

"A hundred years ago, the chemical industry was terrible about protecting us from chemicals that kill cells. Now we're dealing with chemicals that disrupt cellular development, chemicals that interact with DNA and may cause mutations that can lead to cancer. The stakes of not dealing with endocrine disrupters are very high. We need to address endocrine disrupters from inside chemistry." It all comes back to chemical design, Collins believes.

"The body has a magnificent mechanism for destroying chemicals," says Collins. And some chemicals need to be persistent. "Drugs must be persistent to work. But when they get into rivers and lakes—what does that mean over the long term?" Yet, he points out—alluding to the endocrine-disrupting compounds found in so many personal care products, cosmetics, gadgets, and textiles—persistent compounds are being used to "gloss up the life of adults while messing up the life of kids. There needs to be a mandate of intergenerational responsibility in a way we've never seen before."

"There's a fracture in the world of research, with research threatening the status quo of corporate culture. Real-time profits are going to be challenged and it's extremely threatening to certain segments of corporate culture," says Collins. "How do you respond to a new product when there is a problem? Do you pretend it doesn't exist? We need to talk about it publicly. These issues really, really matter, and we need to do something about them."

The morning after a presentation he's given to the Oregon Environmental Council, I have a conversation with Collins over breakfast. "Capitalism can't work for sustainability without credible government constraints," he tells me. "We've been obsessed by technical performance and entirely missed anticipating bioaccumulation."

When I ask how he got interested in what has become the field of green chemistry, Collins talks about a summer he spent in the early 1970s working for a refrigerator manufacturer in New Zealand. "That's when I learned how toxic benzene was," he says. What he discovered was that in the process of sealing the refrigerator liners, hot tar was used. To clean off any hot tar used in sealing the refrigerator liners that splashed on the refrigerators' enamel, workers used rags dipped in solvent. These workers were getting nosebleeds and headaches, which Collins eventually connected with symptoms of exposure to benzene. It turned out the solvent being used was indeed made with benzene and with two related aromatic hydrocarbon compounds, xylene and toluene—both of which are highly toxic.

It was this event—which ended with the frustration of being told by both company chemists and the New Zealand Institute of Chemistry that there was little that could be done—and a case at about the same time of babies in New Zealand born with birth defects, likely as a result of local pesticide spraying, that made Collins became acutely aware of the toxic perils of industrial chemicals.

This concern has stayed with him throughout his career, which includes a 1999 U.S. EPA Presidential Green Chemistry Challenge award for developing what are called "activator chemicals," catalysts that work with hydrogen peroxide to perform industrial tasks traditionally performed by chlorine bleach. These compounds, which Collins's research group at Carnegie Mellon call TAML catalysts, can be used in the wood pulp and paper industry where use of chlorine compounds typically results in waste products that include dioxins. By taking chlorine out of the equation and substituting a compound that breaks down into water and oxygen, a basic hazard is eliminated from the entire process. Perhaps even more significantly, these hydrogen peroxide compounds can be designed to detoxify specific persistent pollutants including organochlorine pesticides, estrogen, and estrogenic compounds.[1] A number of these compounds have been patented by Carnegie Mellon and are now being adapted for industrial use.

These catalysts are "ligands," which Collins explains is simply the name for a grouping of atoms that are placed around a catalytic metal site that conveys particular biochemical and physical properties to that metal. While these compounds can be created through chemical engineering, they also exist in nature. One example of naturally occurring—and critically important—ligands are the enzymes based on iron found in the liver. Their job is to detoxify or break down other compounds that may enter the body. This they do through chemical reactions that result in benign substances—oxygen and water.

"Our catalysts," he says of the ligands his lab has been producing, which are modeled on the liver's detoxification process, "are about 1 percent of the size of natural enzymes, but they're designed to do the same thing. . . . We created equivalent molecules in the laboratory—catalysts that will break larger compounds down to elemental levels." Collins's lab has produced more than twenty TAML ligands so far, Collins tells me. Each one conveys different properties to iron and each creates specific properties that can interact—like enzymes—with specific pollutants to break them down.

These compounds can be used to degrade contaminants that are not removed from municipal water supplies by wastewater treatment plants. Other TAML peroxide compounds remove the dark colors associated with paper production and in the process eliminate the need for and smell associated with organochlorines—that distinctive pulp-mill tang. The fact that these compounds can also prevent dye transfer, Collins explains, means there could be a large benefit in adding small amounts of these catalysts to commercial laundry detergent. If you don't have to worry about dye transfer, there's no reason to separate colors from whites. This ultimately means fewer laundry loads—particularly for commercial laundries but also in the textile industry—and thus less use of both energy and water. These catalysts can destroy most oxidizable things—compounds that can be broken down chemically with oxygen—in water so they are "revolutionary in terms of what it can do for cleaning water," says Collins of his TAML compounds.

"They're not commercially available yet," says Collins, "but we've started to make commercial quantities. We have done fairly major field trials—and done detailed mechanistic studies in the lab. But from an environmental point of view, I don't want to have any nasty surprises further down the road, so we're very careful about watching the degradation all they way down, keeping a close eye on the toxicity as we go," he says.

The effort to eliminate hazardous chemicals "will be no easy ride," Collins wrote in an op-ed for the *Pittsburgh Post-Gazette* in 2008. "We have been part of the way before, but we have ceded much of the landscape to industry 'highwaymen' who would prefer to keep the status quo with toxic chemicals to protect their bottom line." What we need to do, he says, is effectively regulate chemicals that impair development and require that all ingredients on products be listed.[2]

"The right thing is starting to happen throughout the United States and the world on this," says Collins, alluding to growing awareness and restriction of some of these persistent and pervasive compounds. "But it's very contentious," he says. Collins, for one, is not shying away from this engagement. "Green chemistry," he says in his public lectures, "has to be, to some extent, a contact sport," because, as he points out emphatically, "our civilization is not sustainable as currently configured."

⚛ ⚛ ⚛

To find out what's going on where this contact sport of green chemistry is being played, I went to the eleventh annual Green Chemistry & Engineering Conference sponsored by the American Chemical Society, held at the Capital Hilton in Washington, D.C., over several hot, steamy days in late June 2007. Among the hundreds of attendees were representatives of major chemical and pharmaceutical companies, agribusiness conglomerates, NASA, the U.S. Defense Department, academic scientists, consultants and business representatives from around the world, and some nongovernmental organizations that promote sustainable production policies. The PowerPoint presentations were filled with chemical equations and molecular diagrams but the conference atmosphere was oriented more toward business than research science or policy. When I think about this, it makes sense. For what Paul Anastas, Terry Collins, John Warner, and their colleagues are essentially trying to do is sell the petrochemical giants of this world not just a whole new product line but a whole new way of conducting business and measuring product success. And what makes this sales job especially challenging is that for green chemistry to be truly successful, it will mean a shift away from chemical products that, by all historical corporate standards, have performed admirably and generated profits for years—in some cases for generations.

"It's in our best interest to provide leadership toward health and sustainability," says Brad Thompson, president of the plywood and veneer division of Columbia Forest Products at the conference's opening plenary session. According to their calculations, Columbia Forest Products, the largest plywood manufacturer in North America, conversion of all of their plants from producing a layered plywood that uses a urea-formaldehyde-based adhesive to one with a soy-based adhesive would reduce operating emissions here by 50 to 90 percent. It would also save the company money.

"Who would have thought that one could change the hardwood-plywood industry with an adhesive," says Thompson. This revolutionary soy-based adhesive was developed by Dr. Kaichang Li, a research scientist at Oregon State University in collaboration with the Hercules Company, a chemical manufacturer. The adhesive was considered innovative and environmentally friendly enough to win a 2007 Presidential Green Chemistry Challenge Award. The soy-flour-based adhesive, according to Dr. Li, was developed to mimic the workings of the liquid protein that mussels use to attach themselves to rocks. Li analyzed the proteins in both mussel enzymes and soy and developed a process that would render soy proteins capable of the mussel proteins' adhesive properties. This product, called PureBond, is now being produced exclusively by Hercules and used by Columbia Forest Products.

"From a business perspective it's always in our best interest to have healthy customers," says Thompson. "Green chemistry is just plain good business." The soy-based adhesive, Thompson points out, now costs less than the formaldehyde adhesive. What he doesn't mention, I think to myself as I listen to the presentation, are the considerable environmental and health benefits of formally discontinuing use of formaldehyde adhesives in plywood and veneer products altogether and legally barring these wood products in the United States as in other countries. It was, after all, the embalming-fluid levels of formaldehyde, a probable carcinogen, that emanated from paneling in the notorious New Orleans FEMA mobile homes and travel trailers, that prompted lawsuits from families who had been exposed. Why is formaldehyde still in use anywhere, I wonder, if this effective, cost-efficient, and nontoxic alternative that Thompson is using is available?

The soy being used for the commercial production of Dr. Li's mussel-mimicking adhesive is supplied by Cargill, the agribusiness giant. At the conference, Ron Christiansen, Cargill's corporate vice president and chief technology officer, tells us that his company's business "starts at the farm, not at the oil field." Cargill, he says, has a great interest in "adding value to what farmers grow," which means looking for new markets, products, and applications. Among these are plastics. Cargill has apparently been supplying the raw material for corn-based plastics since the late 1980s and is now joint owner, with the Japanese company Teijin, of the biopolymer manufacturer NatureWorks, which manufactures plastics that are based on polylactic acid (PLA) made from dextrose or corn sugar.[3]

This corn-based and biodegradable polymer can now be found as beverage cups, food containers, and fibers that go into both paper and textile products. The versatile polymer is also being used to package batteries and to make clear plastic containers for takeout food, egg cartons, coffee bags, beverage bottles, and what the company calls "tableware."

NatureWorks has customers all around the world, including some large producers and chains like Del Monte Fresh, Subway, 7-Eleven, and Green Mountain Coffee Roasters. There are currently dozens of textile manufacturers listed on NatureWorks's website as suppliers of products using the PLA-based fibers sold under the brand name Ingeo. In addition to these corn-based polymers, Cargill is also making bio-based flexible foam products for use in upholstery, bedding, flooring, and car seats, to mention but a few applications.

These plastics can be recycled and, according to NatureWorks, reusable PLA can be recovered from used PLA plastics. While they are biodegradable, these plastics won't simply dissolve if left out in the rain and apparently do require some real heat and humidity to break down in composting—more than is probably generated by the average backyard compost pile in northern climates.

"The early attempts at bio-based flexible foam literally stunk," says Christiansen. "They smelled bad, like burnt popcorn." (This was true of early soy-based inks as well, which gave off an odor of faintly rancid cooking oil.) But the odor issue was resolved and the result, he claims, is a product that performs favorably compared to petroleum-based products. "Only by creating products that work as well as those based on petroleum will green chemistry succeed," says Christiansen. And, he notes, "profitability needs to be there if we're going to be there too."

Many companies have begun to make additional kinds of bio-based flexible foams—the materials that go into flooring tiles and floor coverings, carpet backing, insulation, upholstery fabrics and padding, and the kinds of moldable plastics used in vehicles, to name just a few examples. What gives these materials their distinctive and varying flexibility are air cells. If you look at a cross-section of any of these materials you'll find tiny—or not so tiny, depending on the foam—cells (as you'd see in a slice of celery or tomato skin) stacked like bricks. The plant-based material for these flexible foam—and other plastic—products may be corn, canola, sunflower seeds, soy, or another bean (castor beans, for example).

These engineered plant materials are also being made into rigid plastics, fibers, detergents, and the emulsions that go into cosmetics and personal care products—what DuPont calls "functional fluids." Cargill, Dow, Archer Daniels Midland, DuPont, BASF, and other big chemical and agribusiness companies are all involved, as are many smaller companies along with manufacturers of products into which these foams and fluids are incorporated.

The list of companies designing and making bio-based plastics is now so long it's not feasible to name them all, but the point to take away is that nonpetroleum plastics have now entered the product mainstream and are no longer aimed solely at stereotypically eco conscious consumers. Virtually all the major chemical and pharmaceutical manufacturers say they have now initiated lines of synthetics based on renewable (nonpetroleum) materials. Dow, for example, has announced an antifreeze for boats and recreational vehicles based on food-grade propylene glycol (a petroleum product, but one with very low toxicity) and plant-based rather than petroleum-based ingredients that will be sold at Wal-Mart.

One of the big hurdles to be overcome in the "greening" of the world of flexible foam is the process that turns a liquid oil—vegetable or otherwise—into the final material. What and who makes this happen are, in industry lingo, called foamers. On its own, no oil—soy, corn, canola, or any other—will magically puff up and create a springy, flexible foam. To achieve the desired cellular structure, a foaming agent is required in addition to the base material. The precise combination of material plus foaming agent plus process, which involves disassembling and reassembling the vegetable oil molecules, is generally proprietary to each chemical manufacturer.

Historically isocyanates, hydrochlorofluorocarbons, and chlorofluoro-carbons have been used along with other petroleum derivatives. As HCFCs and CFCs were phased out because of their ozone-depletion properties, isocyanates and other petrochemical foaming agents have dominated the market. Isocyanates exist in many formulas. Among those used in foaming applications include toluene diisocyanate and methyl isocyanate. Both are serious respiratory toxicants and skin irritants, and both are suspected carcinogens. Repeated exposure can lead to asthma-like attacks, pneumonia symptoms, and other breathing problems and in some instances can cause more serious illness or death. In fact, the chemical involved in the deadly 1984 industrial accident in Bhopal, India, was methyl isocyanate.[4] Methyl isocyanate is also the chemical involved in the deadly August 2008 explosion at the Bayer CropScience plant in West Virginia, a plant with a history of chemical leaks.

The current crop of bio-based, flexible foam products are being made with a range of foaming agents, which vary by final product application. Some are being made with carbon dioxide, nitrogen, and water-based agents. But others are manufactured using well-known high-hazard chemicals, including isocyanates and other petrochemicals. The dilemma of "greening" the entire production process, however, is not confined to flexible foams. Currently, there are hazardous chemicals—reagents and solvents—being used to process any number of renewable, bio-based materials.

Pharmaceuticals are among these products, yet they are another area of chemical manufacturing in which green chemistry is beginning to make a few inroads. The resources at present that go into making pharmaceuticals and the waste created in manufacturing them far exceed the physical size and quantity of the finished product (and thereby contributes to high drug costs), according to Joe Fortunak, another presenter at the Green Chemistry conference.

"Big pharma's job," says Fortunak, a professor of pharmaceutical sciences at Howard University who also works with the University of Alabama's Center for Green Manufacturing, "is to create new medicines. And to make what's essential as accessible as possible while making it sustainable. Currently," he says, "about 1 billion people in the world have real access to medicine. Roughly 5.5 billion of the world's 6.5 billion people have inadequate access to medicine." The huge discrepancy stems in part, he suggests, from not only how pharmaceuticals are made but also where they are made. In many African countries, for example, it's too expensive to buy drugs from big pharma: "Sustainable implies equitable access to the fruits of technology. This is why green chemistry has a tremendous opportunity to be accepted in Africa and other places where manufacturing capacity is being built for the first time." I will hear this from other green chemistry advocates as well—that interest in green chemistry curricula is currently much higher in what are traditionally considered developing countries than it is yet in the United States.

Fortunak is here to talk about the potential of a promising plant-based antimalarial drug. This drug and the treatment associated with it is known as artemisinin combination therapy (artemisinin on its own does not work as an antimalarial drug) or ACT. The base ingredient of this treatment, artemisinin, can be extracted from a plant called *Artemsisia annua*, also known as sweet wormwood. The process of extracting artemisinin from plants in a pharmaceutically useful form is slow, so this compound is also now being produced synthetically. What typically happens is that the raw material is exported for processing and manufacture and the final product—the antimalarial drug—is sold back into the low-income countries where the antimalarials are needed, usually at a premium price.

What should happen instead, Fortunak argues, is for the drug to be manufactured in the countries where it will be used. The economic, environmental, and social benefits are many and obvious. One of the goals, says Fortunak, is to eventually simplify synthesis of the drug. "The simpler the synthesis, the smaller the investment [in training, infrastructure, materials], which increases the capacity to expand manufacturing," and to locate production close to where it's most needed. Green chemistry could go a long way toward achieving both goals.

One of the particular steps in the typical pharmaceutical production process most in need of both simplification and a green chemistry transformation—and which is currently a high-cost step both financially and environmentally—is the use of non-water-based solvents and reagents, compounds that are usually petrochemical derivatives, highly toxic, and expensive. Efforts are underway to use forms of carbon dioxide, titanium dioxides, and other oxygen- and water-based compounds to produce desired results, but this part of the metaphorical hazardous and petrochemical aircraft carrier has yet to make a full turn toward green chemistry.

✥ ✥ ✥

Two other areas where green chemistry researchers are hard at work—cosmetics and electronics—may seem poles apart, but they have some surprising similarities—as illustrated by the work of Amy Cannon, an energetic researcher with the Warner Babcock Institute for Green Chemistry and cofounder and executive director of its associated educational nonprofit, the BeyondBenign Foundation. Cannon's work focuses on electronics, specifically formulating environmentally benign chemicals for use in semiconductor and solar-cell production. Development of "green" chemicals for cosmetics, however, has emerged as a sideline thanks to the curious gallery of overlapping polymer applications—and the musings of inquisitive graduate students.

Cannon holds the world's first PhD in green chemistry, which she earned at the University of Massachusetts–Lowell where she worked with John Warner, to whom she is now married. When I first met Cannon in the fall of 2006, I immediately thought how different my college science education might have been if molecular structure had been explained to me by someone with her sunny smile, ebullient enthusiasm, and ability to describe complex chemical materials and processes in easy-to-visualize contextual and narrative terms. While her manner is easy, Cannon's chemistry is serious. She has worked as a consultant for Rohm and Haas, a company that makes specialty chemicals for the electronics industry, and as an analytic chemist for the Gillette Company. She's also taught green chemistry at the University of Massachusetts and now, in addition to her work with Warner Babcock, coordinates the new green chemistry program at Cambridge College in Lawrence, Massachusetts.

"There are," says Cannon, "amazing similarities between the materials used in electronics and cosmetics." Both involve compounds that create flexible, waterproof films and coatings. Historically, the chemicals used to create materials with these properties have been hazardous. Semiconductor photoresists have often involved the use of the perfluorinated chemicals PFOS and PFOA, while many cosmetics have been formulated with polymers that use phthalates to achieve the flexible films that make products like nail polish and mascara adhere to and bend with curved surfaces. Instead of relying on materials with adverse environmental and health impacts to create these properties, Cannon asks: "Can we design a better molecule to begin with?"

"Can we build in the desired function [to the molecule we're designing] but decrease the number of overall molecules we need and so cut down on waste and process steps?" she asks. This idea is at the heart of green chemistry. Instead of forcing molecules to do something they wouldn't on their own, green chemistry tries to build function into the new molecule's design, Cannon explains.

The chemical films typically used as photoresist materials in semiconductor production are designed to work on a substrate—the surface onto which the circuitry pattern is etched—silicon wafers, for example. After a pattern is carved onto the surface by exposing the photoresist polymer to light, the resist is removed with a solvent, leaving the etched pattern behind. Traditionally, this etching has been done with what Cannon describes as "very active, very toxic, very small molecules" and through a multistep process that uses lots of hazardous solvents. Chemicals in semiconductor production have, over the years, exposed thousands of workers to toxic chemicals—sometimes with tragic results—and have resulted in millions of pounds of hazardous chemical effluent and emissions. Cannon simply asks: "Can we do this better?"

In one of her lectures, Cannon explains how she worked on special technical materials used in laptops and other portable high-tech electronics. "We had all sorts of design criteria for new products," she says. "Things had to have a certain solubility, a specific melting point, certain mechanical properties—strength and flexibility—a certain refractive index, and a specific surface tension. We'd talk about all of this in great detail then I'd ask, 'What about the toxicity? What about the environmental impact?' We were just told to look for performance criteria without any reference to toxicity or environmental impact."

Safety, says Cannon, can be thought of as just another property of a material. The materials we design, she says, must perform as well as or better than the alternatives, be environmentally benign, and be more economical than alternatives. One of these goals without the others is not really what she's after.

As Cannon explains it, what green chemistry is trying to do is design molecules that work the way they do in nature. This is how the soy-based adhesive that can replace formaldehyde in plywood came about. This is also where some of the allure of nanotechnology lies—in creating new molecules by taking advantage of natural attractions and chemical reactions, exploiting their ability to assemble, disassemble, and reassemble without the use of excess force or heat, either applied physically or in the form of chemical reagent. To achieve this in the realm of semiconductor production—a complex, multistep process that now involves dozens of hazardous chemicals—would be revolutionary.

"I always wanted to save the world," Cannon says about her path to green chemistry. "We heard about all the environmental problems," she says, "but far less about solutions." In college her focus in chemistry was on environmental issues and that included an analysis of mercury in fish—mercury pollution being a problem throughout New England, where she grew up. Later, in graduate school, she ended up working on her master's degree as part of John Warner's new green chemistry group at the University of Massachusetts–Lowell. And while not one of the best places to work if, as Cannon put it, "you have an environmental conscience," she's worked as an analytical chemist creating specialty materials for major manufacturing companies, experience she values.

Some of the polymers Cannon has been working with as a green chemist were discovered by trying to create a material whose molecular design enables it to, in effect, be multifunctional—and thereby eliminate extraneous steps and extra materials. Among these materials is a polymer based on thymine, a constituent of the compounds that make up the nucleic acids in DNA. Thymine turns out to be even more multipurpose than she and her colleagues initially imagined. Not only can it be used to make semiconductors, it can also be used in a beauty salon.

Thymine is a big molecule and what Cannon calls a "preformed polymer." If you shine light on it, it crosslinks—connects or bonds—and creates a polymer. This is how thymine often works in the human body. If UV light hits thymine molecules, it produces a kink in the DNA that triggers what Cannon calls "a little enzyme repair mechanism." This reaction sends a signal that says some crosslinking needs to be done. (The inspiration for this choice of molecule, Cannon explains, came from the UV light treatment John Warner underwent for psoriasis in which faulty cells are prompted to repair themselves through light exposure.)

She and her colleagues created a thymine compound with molecular sites that are available for polymerization—or crosslinking. They were able to build a variety of polymers this way, including some that are water soluble. They also discovered that the addition of another enzyme (one found in *E. coli*) can "unzip" the polymer so that the original thymine building blocks are recoverable and ostensibly available for reuse.

The thymine polymer Cannon and her colleague created turns out to be quite versatile. It can be tinted with food color dye, giving it possibilities for consumer product applications. These polymers can be turned into time-release systems by controlling how densely polymerized the material is and thus can be used in drug delivery or to encapsulate pharmaceuticals that need to dissolve over a specified time period. The thymine polymer can also be given a coating that resists bacteria. "Bacteria won't grow on this surface," says Cannon, eliminating the need for antibacterial additives (many currently used have proven to be persistent pollutants). It can also be used in the application for which it was originally developed, in photoresists for electronics.

It also turns out that this polymer can literally make your hair curl. As Cannon tells the story, she and John Warner were having lunch with some students and conversation somehow got around to discussing the viscosity of Dippity Do hair gel. This prompted the students to return to the lab, put the thymine polymer on some hair, curl the strands, and expose them to UV light. The result: the curls stayed put. The experiment found its way into a PowerPoint presentation, which Cannon and Warner happened to mention while meeting with a corporation about a technical commercial application for the thymine cross-polymer. The company—Cannon doesn't name it—happens to have a personal care products division and the executives were deeply impressed with the prospect of a nontoxic permanent wave product. This might seem like a joke, but as Cannon explains, the current methods used for chemically perming and straightening hair involve highly toxic substances and processes.

Cosmetics may seem trivial in the great scheme of things, but they are a widespread source of multiple chemical exposures for millions of people, including pregnant women. Cosmetics, Cannon notes, are not overseen by either the FDA or the EPA, so their overall product safety is actually poorly regulated. A nontoxic perm might not be on a par with curing cancer but it would change the lives of the thousands of women who work with and use these cosmetics products.

Among such products are nail polishes. Historically nail polish has been formulated with toxic ingredients, among them formaldehyde, toluene, phthalates, and acetone. The result, particularly for beauty salon workers, is substantial chemical exposures. The University of Massachusetts–Lowell's Toxics Use Reduction Institute (TURI) has been working with local beauty and nail salons to reduce use of hazardous materials and thereby improve conditions for workers as well as customers.

"This seems to be a miracle product," Cannon says laughingly of the thymine polymer. "So we said, why not try it on our nails." Because the thymine compound binds easily to food-grade dyes, and because nail polishes are basically photoresists, Cannon and colleagues experimented by attaching a blue-green dye to the polymer. They then painted it on a nail-substitute surface and exposed it to light. The green water-soluble polymer successfully coated the surface, demonstrating that this compound has the potential to create a nontoxic nail polish. Not only is the potential polish nontoxic but it can be removed with an enzyme wash that's also nontoxic rather that the hazardous acetone and other volatile organic solvents typically used to remove nail polish. And since the polymer takes dye and works on hair, why not try developing a nontoxic hair dye, suggests Cannon. "Although you may not want blue hair," she laughs.

Cannon and her group are working to make the polymer work at light wave lengths that are safer for people than those used in the initial experiments, something that would extend the polymer's application. They are also looking into using a bio-based, biodegradable substrate, including one based on potatoes, to "get away from the politics of corn," says Cannon. For Cannon's lab, potatoes also have the advantage of being relatively local—initiatives are now underway in Maine to develop polylactic acid using locally grown potatoes.

Ultimately, what makes this thymine polymer so innovative is that rather than offering a drop-in substitution for an objectionable ingredient, it in effect rethinks the entire concept of a functional material by linking synthesis and function. Rather than relying on additives to make a material perform the desired function, the material itself can be designed to do everything needed, and in this case it can do so without being toxic or persistent. Yet because nearly everything currently on cosmetics counters, drugstore shelves, and in electronics factories relies on the petrochemicals we've been using for decades, it may take a while—and more consumer demand—before materials like Amy Cannon's become the norm.

❖ ❖ ❖

To get an idea of how interest in green chemistry might be moving out of the laboratory and into the marketplace, I sat down over coffee in Somerville, Massachusetts, with Mark Rossi, research director of Clean Production Action, a nonprofit that advocates for environmentally preferable, nontoxic products. Because the word "green" is now slapped on just about any product imaginable and there's no real way to know exactly what it means, Clean Production Action has been working to create what Rossi calls a "green screen": a way to assess whether a chemical material is environmentally benign and without adverse human health impacts. Astonishingly enough, despite acres worth of databases maintained by government agencies, industries, academic sources, and nongovernmental organizations that are available to anyone with access to a computer and an Internet search engine, this information is still frustratingly obscure, incomplete, confusing, and sometimes misleading.

The different U.S. agencies that deal with chemical safety issues—among them the EPA, the Centers for Disease Control, OSHA, and NIOSH—frequently offer different toxicity assessments for the same substance. Not only do safety standards (safe exposure levels) differ from agency to agency—and from state to state—but the assessment of health effects can also differ as well. Some of these databases are astonishingly out of date, in some cases by decades.[5] Different databases under the same agency umbrella sometimes contain different data; some contain few data at all even about substances that are now well studied. The upshot is that it's extremely difficult to know which of the many supposedly unbiased government sources offers the most reliable or currently accurate information, leaving the criteria of "safe" very much in limbo.

A vast database that is supposed to help provide chemical users—professional rather than casual public users—with information on the thousands of chemicals produced in or imported to the United States at high commercial volume is the High Production Volume Information System (HPVIS). Its current iteration was rolled out in December 2006, just about the same time that the European Union was passing its new chemical safety legislation known as REACH (Registration Evaluation, and Authorization of Chemicals). In a number of ways, the debate around what the U.S. HPVIS program does or does not do, and why, is the backstory to the work of Rossi's group and others advocating for U.S. chemical policy reform. The limited usefulness of the HPVIS program and other current chemical safety databases for improving environmental health also illustrate, I think, why continuing to address chemical safety on a chemical-by-chemical basis without addressing chemical and materials safety from the molecular design and hazard-removal perspective, we're unlikely to solve current pollution problems.

The details of the HPVIS program—which was created with substantial input from the American Chemistry Council, the American Petroleum Institute and, at the other end of the interest-group spectrum, the Environmental Defense Fund—are fairly mind-numbing. But the bottom line is that participation in the registry is voluntary and lacks any regulatory or enforcement power. Although the EPA does issue nonbinding "challenges" or calls for information, it relies on information provided by manufacturers (rather than on third-party testing) and it requires no new testing of chemicals if data for the requested environmental and health effects are available.[6] One so-called "endpoint" of toxicity not included, however, is endocrine disruption, and as Richard Dennison, senior scientist for the Environmental Defense Fund has pointed out, the environmental and health testing effects currently in the HPVIS program were developed twenty or more years ago.[7]

The requirements of the HPVIS program differ notably from those of the European Union's REACH legislation. While the American program is voluntary, REACH is mandatory. Under REACH, the toxicity data that must be provided on all chemicals produced or used at volumes over 1 metric ton (2,200 pounds) annually include endocrine disruption as one of its testing criteria. REACH requires manufacturers to prepare substitution plans for substances deemed of very high toxicity concern. It also has a provision to cover what it calls "substances in articles," chemicals that can be expected to be released from consumer products—synthetic fragrances, for example. (In contrast, some U.S. chemical manufacturers talk about measuring "cradle-to-gate" impacts of their products, meaning that their assessment ends when the product leaves the factory, in effect ignoring impacts—possibly harmful—that may arise during normal product use, disposal, or recycling.) Chemical products not registered with the REACH program, furthermore, cannot be exported to the EU. As of 2008, REACH was expected to involve registration of about 30,000 chemicals and eventually to result in the ban or restriction of some 1,500 chemicals.

The HPVIS program also raises the questions of quantity of information versus quality of information and how effectively this program can be used to protect environmental health. "If we wait until a chemical reaches high production volume to trigger this kind of data, it means the substance is already a very important one to the economy," says Michael Wilson, a research scientist in the Center for Occupational and Environmental Health at the University of California Berkeley's School of Public Health.[8] This also means that in addition to substantial financial investments in such materials, there will have been ample opportunity for people to be exposed to this substance either during manufacturing or at any other point in the product's life. But even the amount of documentation seems subject to debate, as evidenced by the statement from the American Chemistry Council in response to passage of REACH: "The ACC believes that the European Commission's . . . [REACH] proposal seeks considerably more information than required by regulatory authorities to assure that chemicals are produced and used as safely as possible. REACH is unworkable, impractical, and costly—and will not provide the health and environmental benefits envisioned by its creators."[9]

REACH does represent a significant step toward requiring manufacturers to provide toxicity information on their products and ensure their safety prior to commercialization. It also has the regulatory power to restrict them under a system that puts the burden of proof of safety on the manufacturer rather than the burden of proving harm on the consumer as does the United States's Toxic Substances Control Act (TSCA).

"From where we sit, the public is increasingly questioning the safety of chemicals in the products they use and purchase," said Gary Gulka of the Vermont Department of Environmental Conservation at that 2006

EPA meeting, describing increasing state interest in environmentally preferable purchasing and green chemistry. This is where Mark Rossi's Clean Production Action group comes in. "Right now," says Rossi, "data cut both ways for the environmental community. We need data on both existing chemicals and safer substitutes, but the lack of either can be an argument for continuing with the use of a known substance." And, Rossi adds, "Just because it's 'natural' doesn't mean it's not toxic."

•ᐧ• •ᐧ• •ᐧ•

Our current approach to environmental health protection is not holistic and still centers around what can be achieved with individual chemical bans or restrictions. This focus continues to be the typical of regulations at the state, local, and federal levels in the United States. This holds true for the 2008 Consumer Product Safety Improvement Act, which while covering a range of products—including children's products in which it restricts lead and half a dozen phthalates—does so by focusing on specific chemicals rather than classes of comparable chemicals and includes no programmatic provisions for developing alternative products. A few exceptions to this approach have recently emerged, and green chemistry advocates hope these will prompt more systemic improvements in materials safety and environmental health protection.

Among the most notable of these exceptions was a program announced in May 2007 by the state of California. Called the "Green Chemistry Initiative," the program aims to move beyond chemical-by-chemical restrictions and shift to a more proactive pollution prevention policy by solving toxicity problems at the design stage and by replacing hazardous substances currently in use with safer alternatives. Policy advocates at the nonprofit organization Environment California are generally supportive of the initiate's aims and first steps, but point out that the program currently lacks sufficient regulatory provisions and that to be effective it needs information about chemical products that manufacturers are not yet required to disclose. A similarly notable exception is the Michigan Green Chemistry Program created by executive order by Governor Jennifer Granholm in 2006. Its aim is to coordinate research and development of new environmentally benign chemicals and products within Michigan and is seen as a way to help revitalize the state's manufacturing industries.

Although not explicitly a green chemistry bill, in January 2008, the Massachusetts state senate passed "An Act for a Healthy Massachusetts: Safer Alternatives to Toxic Chemicals." Also known simply as the Safer Alternatives bill, the law would set up a program to identify chemicals that pose a "significant risk to human health or the environment" and to make recommendations for safe alternatives. As of April 2009, the bill had yet to pass the legislature in full. Other states, including Connecticut, Maine, Illinois, Michigan, Vermont, Alaska, and New York, have also been considering legislation that goes beyond chemical-by-chemical restrictions, either by promoting green chemistry efforts, advancing environmentally preferable purchasing programs, or with bills that target toxics in children's products.

A great many more states have also been working on bills that would restrict the use of certain specific chemicals such as bisphenol A, certain brominated flame retardants, phthalates, and perfluorinated chemicals along with various pesticides, lead, and mercury. Most of the legislation that would bar use of specific chemicals, however, has been opposed by chemical industries, as have the more comprehensive bills. Ironically, some of the chemical manufacturing companies that have spent money to lobby against these policies are at the same time investing substantially in efforts to develop environmentally preferable alternatives to their own hazardous products.

Despite the piecemeal and often contentious nature of regulation and legislation, many manufacturing companies whose products depend on synthetic chemicals are shifting their chemical choices to nontoxics well ahead of—and with a speed that exceeds—passage of any regulation or legislation, notes Lara Sutherland of the nonprofit Health Care Without Harm. Such efforts are going on worldwide both in commercial, industrial and academic research with applications that range from energy production to textiles and packaging.

While discontinuing the use of one material in favor of another does not necessarily constitute green chemistry, the need to do so—for example, when prompted by restriction of a hazardous material—may well prompt innovation. Being able to offer a new product, especially one that will work as well as or better than the existing one, rather than an empty shelf when a new regulation goes into effect is the challenge—and why manufacturers are so keen to stay well ahead of the regulatory curve. What's been happening with polyvinyl chloride (PVC) is a case in point. PVC contains phthalates—the plasticizers that are coming under increasing scrutiny and regulation because of their adverse health impacts—and when burned, as it will be if disposed of in municipal incinerators or many rudimentary landfills or dumps, PVC releases persistent and extremely toxic dioxins and furans. So while PVC is not legally restricted anywhere, many manufacturers, alert to growing public and scientific concern, are moving to other materials.

There already are some other packaging materials that perform comparably to PVC, but many companies have also begun to shift away from PVC as a structural material. Electronics companies, including HP, Dell, and Lenovo have 2009 as the date by which PVC will eliminated from packaging and products. Apple has already discontinued PVC packaging and other applications with the exception of some external wiring, and Microsoft stopped using PVC packaging in 2005. It's important to note that none of these companies actually makes PVC, packaging materials, or wire cables, so this kind of product redesign involves people up and down the supply chain. Nike also has a PVC phaseout underway. Meanwhile, on the retail side of the equation, Wal-Mart, Target, Sears, Kmart, Toys "R" Us, along with toy manufacturers Mattel and Hasbro, among others, are discontinuing sales of toys made with PVC.[10]

Sony has gone even further in altering its plastics use. Having eliminated PVC from packaging and product cases, it has begun to use bio-based plastics for its electronics. For example, the company is already using castor-oil based polymers in cameras, DVD players, and its Walkman MP3 players among other products that include a "smart" card (notable simply because there are so many of these pieces of plastic about).

When it comes to finding alternatives to PVC in applications other than packaging—such as in screen-printing, a technique used to apply team insignia on sports gear, for example—eliminating PVC means not just finding an alternative material with comparable performance, but redesigning the entire process. As a Nike executive explained to me, no team wants to be the one on the field wearing shirts with their name peeling off. Eric Beckman, professor of engineering at the University of Pittsburgh, characterizes this performance problem by noting that people want "things that are both stable and unstable at the same time." We want the durability provided by a PVC but for environmental reasons, want materials that will biodegrade.

Nike has also been rethinking its use of solvents and adhesives. Those in longest, widest use often involve volatile organic compounds (VOCs), typically substances based on benzene and chlorine chemistry. Phasing out these toxics is not a straightforward substitution. The switch to aqueous, non-VOC-based glues and solvents has in some cases meant changing the whole production process. With one product, I was told, the old VOC-based adhesive dried quickly. Using a water-based adhesive meant increasing the time the pieces had to be physically held until dry, increasing the overall production time. "Where you were making a hundred pieces in a set period of time, you might now be making seventy," I was told. To meet the previous production rate, other parts of the process or product would also have to be redesigned. But such changes are achievable. For example, in 2004 Nike was using less than 5 percent of the VOCs per pair of shoes manufactured than it used in 1995. Similarly, the majority of the rubber Nike now uses in its footwear is made with only 4 percent of the chemicals it had identified as used in these materials prior to 1994.[11]

"We are at an inflection point of unprecedented historical development," Mark Wysong, CEO of Dolphin Safe Source, a consulting company that works with businesses—including *Fortune* 500 companies—to reduce their use of toxic chemicals, said optimistically in 2007. A survey of 4,000 professionals had found that about one-third considered reduction of toxic chemicals among the top three the most important environmental issues, ranking behind only global warming and energy conservation.

"Today there are more than 100,000 such chemicals used in more than 3 million products. There were almost none in the early 1930s," notes

Wysong. He also points out that many separate chemicals are often used where far fewer would work as well. This redundancy means that it may actually be easier than a company thinks to reduce overall chemical use. In recent years, says Wysong, General Motors and Delta Airlines each reported about a 30 percent reduction in their chemical use, while Wal-Mart had eliminated about thirty hazardous chemicals from its supply chain. He also notes that to assess its chemical use a company often needs to change perspective. As an example, Wysong described a company that uses one chemical glass cleaner. It's only one chemical, so overall chemical exposure to the company is small. But the cleaner is used every day by the same two janitors; for those workers, the exposure is huge.

❖ ❖ ❖

"We have one goal," says Earl Brown, a lawyer with the American Center for International Labor Solidarity, "and that is to drive up the cost of human life and human labor in Asia, where it is simply far too cheap." I'm sitting in a room with representatives of organizations based in Thailand, India, China, the Philippines, Taiwan, Vietnam, California, Indonesia, Nepal, Bangladesh, Cambodia, Japan, Korea, Malaysia, France, Hong Kong, Australia, and Canada. Their organizations work for the people whom the world regularly forgets—the people behind the pallet loads and shipping containers filled with the cheap goods we all gobble up. These are the people at the far end of the supply chain whose lives could be vastly improved if green chemistry were the universal norm.

We are shown pictures of men in Indonesia handling powdered asbestos, putting it into name-brand motorcycle brake-pads that will be sold all around the world. These men work without protective gloves or masks. In mines, quarries, and other job sites around Asia workers continue to breathe silica dust and suffer from lung disease. I meet colleagues of women who make cadmium-based batteries. Some of these women have suffered miscarriages while others have had babies with birth defects and babies who are always ill. A Malaysian woman who works in the electronics industry describes how women there in their thirties are being given voluntary retirement packages, in her view to encourage the already high worker turnover rate. Many of her coworkers over the years have suffered chronic illnesses but it's been impossible to link them definitively to anything in the factories because of the high turnover rate and lack of monitoring. We also hear from accident victims and their colleagues struggling to receive adequate compensation and medical coverage for their injuries. These stories are not "breaking news" but the lingering realities of the world's far-flung global supply chain. It's also a vivid illustration of how eliminating hazard will eliminate risk and avoid a litany of costly adverse impacts.

Some of this work under hazardous labor conditions is going on not far from where this group of labor and environmental activists has gathered in the Kowloon district of Hong Kong. To get a glimpse, I take an hour's high-speed ferry ride to Shekou, the eastern port for Shenzen, China, and now the third largest port in Asia. It's late August, oppressively hot, bright, and humid. The ferry zips away from the skyscrapers lining Hong Kong's shoreline, past steep green hills characteristic of the South China Sea, and past the new bridges with spans that look like pale piano wires or a professional egg-slicer. The Outlying Islands stretch out to the east in the hot, white-blue light.

The ship traffic, some months before the worldwide recession sets in, across the open harbor waters of the Pearl River Delta looks like rush hour at Times Square. I've never seen so much working boat traffic. Barges piled high with semi-truck sized, cobalt blue and barn red shipping containers emblazoned with the names of freight giants—Haijin, Maersk, China Shipping, Zealand—cross paths with cranes, dredges, and ferries. In between are smaller boats that bring the word scow to mind, their wooden hulls rimmed with tire bumpers underneath three-sided cabins with shallow curved black roofs. On the shoreline of one harbor island, planted on a pile of big beige riprap rocks, in the broiling sun, is someone under an umbrella with a fishing line.

This is one of the world's most notoriously polluted river mouths. It's here that effluent from the industries of Guangdong Province pools. The bulk of these factories are now farther inland, near Guangzhou and points north. But significant levels of perfluorinated chemicals, brominated flame retardants, bisphenol A, PCBs, and other dioxin-like chemicals have been found here as well as in people living and working throughout the region. Of course none of this is visible on the choppy surface of the celadon-green water or in the hazy air. But the acres of city-block-high piles of shipping containers attest to the volume of manufacturing.

Edward Chan of Greenpeace China takes me on a tour of some Shenzhen neighborhoods filled with small factories. The city is a maze of new high-rises and dispiriting old industrial buildings and adjacent dormitory-style apartment blocks. The few people out in the midday sun carry umbrellas for shade, even while cycling. We drive beneath the smokestacks of an asphalt plant and a glass factory. Black plumes of smoke dissipate into the haze. We veer away from the sleek buildings bearing the insignia of world-famous electronics brand names, away from clean plate glass windows and shopping plazas where office workers in white shirts and men in sweaty work clothes line up at ATMs. We head for gray warrens of cement-block buildings where the residences are distinguished from manufacturing facilities by laundry. Balconies are draped with blue and orange smocks, rows of gray limp T-shirts, and faded undershorts. A large portion of Shenzhen's population are not official city residents, Edward tells me. They live here temporarily to work, hence the dormitory-style housing.

Edward and I get out and walk around underneath belching exhaust fans, dripping drainpipes, rattling metal vents, and open work areas, some barred by gates. "What are they making here?" I ask as we pass whirring machinery and look into dim interiors where workers in smocks and coveralls turn to eye us warily. "Plastic parts. Plastics. Pens and pencils. Boxes and envelopes. Plastics," Edward tells me. Some of the exhaust fans and hose pipes face the balconies where laundry is drying only a few feet away.

There are banners everywhere with big bright characters. Here and there I see "ISO1400" and "ROHS." I ask Edward to translate. The signs proclaim compliance with environmental standards and honor the health and safety of the workers. The heat- and soot-laden air compares only to a New York City subway platform on the hottest of summer days. To spell us from the industrial exhaust, we walk along a city river. I look down at the water and hope I'm seeing the dirtiest river I'll ever see. The surface is mottled black and oil-slick blue. There is raw sewage. There are dead and bloated rodents. There is food waste and plastic debris. And there is grimy water pouring from some sort of outfall drainage. Edward urges me to take a video of a particularly foul stream of effluent. Our driver, who's wearing wraparound sunglasses and a black Nike T-shirt, and whose spotless black sedan suggests a clientele other than freelance journalists and environmental activists, seems perplexed by our tour route.

At the station where we catch the bus back to Kowloon is a pair of trash cans—one yellow, one green—that say in English (and presumably Cantonese), "Love our homeland" and "Environmental protection." That evening in Hong Kong, I take a walk down Nathan Road past dozens of electronics stores, shops filled with watches, trendy clothes, and accessories. To cool off I step into an air-conditioned department store where I find myself surrounded by costume jewelry and children's toys, and I realize I'll never look at small plastic objects the same way again. Looking at all this merchandise and thinking about all those hundreds of shipping containers, I think about what a daunting challenge it is to shift our current materials stream. Putting the merits of overflowing toy boxes and ephemeral accessories aside, I also think how people's lives would change if making such things did not mean fouling rivers and damaging cells.

Virtually every major company now has some sort of sustainability initiative in place. How deep these programs go, whether they address core products or stop at the low-hanging fruit, is a valid question. "Every step in this direction is a good thing," says Brendan Condit of the Organic Exchange, an organization working to promote use of organic cotton as a way to decrease pesticide impacts worldwide. "You do what you can do, what you can sell the board on, and what you can make money on," he tells me, recounting his organization's efforts.[12] I also think back to what Paul Anastas told me: "Perfect should not be the enemy of the excellent."

Many manufacturing companies—the cleaning-product giant SC Johnson, for example—have chosen to work along the lines of what Mark

Rossi and colleagues at Clean Production Action call "green screens." These programs identify priorities, both for chemicals targeted for elimination and reduction and for guiding principles. A number of cleaning products manufacturers—including SC Johnson—are also working with the U.S. EPA's Design for the Environment program, which includes templates for screening two major categories of such product ingredients: surfactants (generally the agents that make things sudsy, soapy, foamy, and emollient) and solvents. This program is being used to develop a list of environmentally benign, nontoxic ingredients from which manufacturers can choose. According to the EPA, about 300 manufacturers are now participating in this program. SC Johnson says that moving to environmentally benign ingredients and products has not cost them money or business.

Sony calls its hazardous chemical priority list, which focuses on chemicals used in both exterior and interior components along with packaging, a "green book." As of April 2008, Sony's Green Book included 18,000 monitored materials. In order to keep track of these materials, Sony must communicate this information and verify use of these substances with its suppliers, of which there are at least 4,000. Adopting the green chemistry principle of "atom economy"—using fewer different substances to achieve functional ends with the goal of zero waste and byproducts—would clearly simplify what a company like Sony has to do to monitor its materials.

Another example of "green screening" programs comes from the largest manufacturer of modular carpeting, InterfaceFLOR, which has what it calls a "Mission Zero" initiative. This program targets waste, fibers, dyes, adhesives, and textile additives and sets the goal of eliminating any associated negative environmental impacts by 2020. Even to begin this process the company has had to "completely redesign processes and materials," says Connie Hersh, InterfaceFLOR's director of sustainable research chemicals and processes. In addition to setting out its own goals and designs, the company has had to collaborate with suppliers and obtain a complete disclosure of all product ingredients, something not typical of business. In short, says Hersh, InterfaceFLOR discovered that to complete its Mission Zero, the company "can't make anything the way we're making it now or with what we're making it now." Number 7 on the company's list of what it calls the "seven fronts of sustainability" is "redesigning commerce."

An important source of support for environmentally benign product lines comes from consortiums of large volume purchasers that are pooling both buying power and information resources for these products. Health care institutions, for example, including many major hospital groups—some working through the organization Health Care Without Harm—are targeting fabrics and plastics in this way. Clearly, there is substantial demand from both institutional and individual consumers, but the definition of what's toxic and what's not keeps changing.

Transparency, too, is still a huge issue. It's still hard from the outside for a consumer to make a clear assessment of what's actually in many manufactured and synthetic chemical products. What labels that proclaim "clean" or "nontoxic" really mean—or what an ingredient listed as "cross-polymer" or "fragrance" contains—is no more well defined than those of breakfast cereals that say, "natural" or "all natural." Chemical regulations in the United States are designed to protect proprietary information, a stumbling block that must be overcome to adequately protect environmental and human health. This was illustrated vividly when I searched the documents the Food and Drug Administration has posted to document its 2008 assessment of bisphenol A. Included in these files were results of various polycarbonate food and beverage containers tested with different substances to measure bisphenol A leaching. Not only were the names of manufacturers of these containers redacted, but in several tests the name of the substance that caused the greatest leaching was blacked out. Clearly there has to be a way to protect public health and avoid scaring people with inconclusive test results without undermining commerce.

As the green chemistry advocates would point out, if we eliminate the hazard to begin with—design materials so that we don't have to quibble and worry endlessly about how much of a biologically active and toxic substance to which we're willing to expose our children and ourselves—

and agree that any such hazards are unacceptable, the issue of redacting files will go away along with the health risks. Right now green chemistry and our evolution to environmentally benign products is in an awkward dance between what we know we don't want and what we would like. The list of chemicals of concern for environmental and health hazards continues to grow as does our knowledge about the impacts of those identified as hazardous and toxic—and we have barely begun to investigate the effects of mixtures of toxic substances, the type of exposure that's a reality for virtually everyone alive today. "It's hard to say we've gotten it all wrong," says Terry Collins, "but the really important generation of green chemists is the next one."

Chemical manufacturers and environmental activists alike can agree that materials that biodegrade into environmentally benign constituents; that do not generate hazardous byproducts during the production process, useful product life, or in recycling and disposal; and that do not cause adverse impacts to human health, wildlife, or the environment at any point in their lifecycle, are ideal. Everyone can also agree that eliminating hazardous waste and adverse environmental and health impacts is ultimately good for business. These goals were summed up by an anecdote recounted by Catherine Hunt, president of the American Chemical Society, who recalled asking students at an international green chemistry conference for their shortest definition of sustainability.[13] Their answer: "It's chemistry that allows us to thrive today without screwing up tomorrow."

EPILOGUE:
REDESIGNING THE FUTURE

The reason to understand a problem is to
empower its solution.
—Paul Anastas

So where do we go from here? Can green chemistry gain the momentum
it needs to effectively and substantively improve the prospects for environmental and human health? Can we reshape the policies we've formulated to deal with chemical hazards to reflect current realities of lifelong
incidental exposure to multiple chemicals—exposure that often begins at
the very earliest stage of development? Can we do this in a way that will
curtail the release of known toxic contaminants, achieve maximum public and environmental health protection, and encourage the design of safe
materials? Can we do this while we still have the resilience to cope with
the impacts of the twentieth century's release of unprecedented biologically active chemical contaminants?

More than forty years ago Rachel Carson warned of a "silent spring."
Twenty years ago, Bill McKibben wrote of the human alteration of every
aspect of the natural world. Nature has not ended, but signs of severe and
subtle disturbance are everywhere. Scientists are now watching natural
systems and cellular feedback loops that have evolved over millennia begin to falter in response to chemical wrenches we've introduced into the
global environment. The materials we've used for the past century have

served us well in many ways. But we can no longer afford—if we ever could—to proceed with designs that serve but one generation.

Making the changes in energy sources and materials that would result even in a "less bad future" for the world's climate and biochemical health, let alone create a new, environmentally benign materials stream, would present enormous challenges in the best of times. In many ways that task has just become more difficult with the precipitous drop in world financial markets in the fall of 2008 and early 2009. Yet it is possible that the juncture at which we find ourselves—environmentally and economically—may provide the impetus we need to reassess and proceed in a new direction.

Skyrocketing gas prices in the summer of 2008 made it easy to envision a future in which we relinquish our dependency on petroleum, a change that would alter both our alarming greenhouse gas emissions and the chemical basis of the majority of our synthetic materials. But as budgets tightened and oil prices dropped there has been a retreat from investments—in technology and human resources—that would make these changes possible. Meanwhile the news coming in from the field continues to show how urgently we need to change the nature of what's being let loose in the environment.

Almost every day brings a new report of additional discoveries about toxic and persistent pollutants and hazards associated with synthetic chemicals—brominated flame retardants and perfluorinated compounds that prompt hyperactivity and induce "deranged" behavior in laboratory mice; waterproofing compounds that appear to increase human infertility; endocrine-disrupting synthetics in common food additives and flooring; dioxins that suppress immune system function; a mix of these chemicals permeating public water supplies where they are feminizing male fish.[1] This is not hyperbole, but a litany of headlines from a single month of new peer-reviewed scientific journal papers published in the first quarter of 2009.

At the same time, atmospheric carbon dioxide levels have climbed well above where they must be to forestall the predicted cascade of ecologically disrupting consequences, including additional release and circulation of persistent pollutants prompted by warming temperatures and exacerbated effects of their impacts. In the fall of 2008, scientists measured the second greatest summer retreat of Arctic Sea ice yet recorded—second only to the previous year's record retreat. This polar ice is now thinner than ever before, a condition that will hasten its melting.[2] Unless we drastically reduce our use of fossil fuels—including coal—say scientists at NASA's Goddard Space Science Institute, these CO_2 levels will continue to rise.[3] Some of the resulting effects may manifest themselves with obvious drama but most are likely to occur with the tempo of a leaky faucet, making it difficult to compel the changes in sources of energy—and therefore materials—that would alter our present course.

There is now substantial evidence that environmental conditions play a role in every complex disease and that environmental pollutants have a profound effect on human health. It is clear that a number of chemicals at levels present in the environment can disrupt genetic programming—the biochemical signals that determine the health of living organisms—in ways that can lead to reproductive, metabolic, immune system, neurological, cardiovascular, pulmonary, and developmental health problems. Some of these effects are irreversible and remain with an individual for life. And some occur at very specific stages of early life with an impact potentially so disruptive that one chemical exposure can affect several generations.

We also know that there are hundreds of synthetic chemicals in use, most of them petroleum-based, that can interfere with vital cellular mechanisms—and more are being discovered every week. Some chemicals recognized as a certain type of toxicant—dioxins for example, long known to be carcinogens—have recently also been shown to have additional adverse health effects, in the case of dioxins, cardiovascular dysfunction, and endocrine disruption. Many of these compounds are used intentionally but many are also present as trace contaminants, as chemical reaction byproducts, or the as result of shoddy or cheap manufacturing.

What makes these omnipresent pollutants particularly problematic is that many of them have been shown to be potentially harmful at incredibly low doses, but we currently regulate primarily at fixed, high doses.

Furthermore, when we do regulate chemicals, we do so one at a time and lack a standard way to assess multiple chemical exposures when it may be the interaction and additive natures of some exposures that is especially harmful.

These substances "are everywhere," says Jerry Heindel, scientific program administrator of the National Institute of Environmental Health Sciences. There are so many of them, "we don't even know where to look next."[4]

❖ ❖ ❖

"We have no choice but to deal with this," Terry Collins has remarked, summing up this state of affairs.[5] It is now clear that our global consumer economy has relied overwhelmingly on materials and energy sources that have proven to be neither environmentally safe nor tenable. And we have moved beyond the point where we had the luxury of postponing significant changes in these materials choices. "Safe technology"—meaning the machines and materials we manufacture—"requires safe energy," notes Collins.

Thus far our efforts to alter this landscape have been incremental and directed toward changing individual materials. While this is successful in some cases, if we're to move beyond dealing with the adverse effects, both immediate and long-term, of manufactured chemicals in what seems like a protracted game of Whac-a-Mole, we need to think about such changes holistically rather than on the basis of drop-in substitutions and lists of individually banned substances. Unless we consider toxicity and hazard on the basis of molecular design and in an ecological context—globally as well as in terms of human health and product ecology—we'll continue to be chasing these problems after they've occurred, a strategy that has proven costly, inefficient, and ultimately insufficiently effective.

For years we've been stuck in a system whose structure has ended up pitting the chemical industry against academic research scientists and nongovernmental environmental health advocates. We have been making environmental health and safety decisions based largely on information supplied by manufacturers about their own products and within a regulatory framework that effectively gives priority to proprietary interests and puts the burden of proof on those who claim harm has been caused.

Compounding the bias implicit in this structure are weaknesses in the Toxic Substances Control Act (TSCA), theoretically our most direct legal vehicle for regulating and taking toxic chemicals off the market. Among the places where TSCA falls down on the job is that exempt from its consideration are substances the manufacturer asserts will have low environmental releases and low human exposure during production, distribution, use, and disposal.[6] Given what we now know about how many hazardous substances enter the world's environment and our bodies—and about the potential effects of low-dose exposures of numerous commercially used synthetic chemicals—this cannot be an effective way to protect environmental health.

TSCA's effectiveness is also hobbled by the provision that the "least burdensome" measures available be used when remedying a situation where manufactured chemicals have caused harm. In practice, "least burdensome" has been taken to mean a remedy that causes the least financial burden to those whose products would be affected—rather than a remedy that would maximize reduction of the burden to those suffering adverse impacts. As currently configured, says Lynn Goldman, professor at the Johns Hopkins Bloomberg School of Public Health and former assistant administrator of the EPA's Office of Pollution Prevention and Toxic Substances, TSCA makes it difficult for the EPA to effectively manage chemicals and results in reliance on unenforceable voluntary measures.[7] This calculus also typically overlooks long term costs to public health and the environment—cost of health care, cost to quality of life, cost of environmental remediation, and cost to fully functioning ecosystems. And, notes Paul Anastas, the protective measures and the endless end-of-pipe solutions into which we continue to pour money "must be a cost drain and cannot add to product performance or to process efficiency."[8]

When considering how to redesign this system, it's important to remember just how many manufactured chemicals we're dealing with. As

Anastas points out, some 3,000 new chemicals are invented or discovered every day. This prodigious activity means that there are now more than 40 million chemicals listed on the American Chemical Society's chemical registry to which about 12,000 new substances are added daily.[9] How and if we'll continue to churn out new compounds at this rate is hard to say but, given the rapid development of nanomaterials, future numbers aside, we're already producing and using hundreds of new materials of novel and largely unknown behavior.

Of these millions of chemicals, explains Anastas, "only 3,112 . . . are recognized by the FDA as active pharmaceutical agents, leaving 99 percent of chemicals other than drugs." This means that the vast majority of synthetic chemicals are not designed with the assumption of any biological activity, leaving us to deal with the discovery of these effects late in the process of chemical synthesis and production—or, as has more often happened, after millions of pounds of a material have gone into consumer products. To prevent perpetuation of similar chemical toxicity problems in the future, we need, says Anastas, "to integrate knowledge of biologically active molecules into the design of non-pharmaceutical synthetics."[10]

Doing so will mean a new vocabulary for synthetic chemists and others who design materials. Performance and price will no longer be the primary considerations for new material viability. Considering biological activity from the beginning of the molecular design process will mean moving away from reliance on the risk analysis central to our current end-of-pipe approach to chemical hazards. By focusing on risk and spending years—in some cases, decades—assessing the extent of that risk, then trying to decide just how much exposure is acceptable and for whom, we've perpetuated the use of countless hazardous substances. With tens of thousands of chemicals in commerce, our current scheme of risk-based chemical regulation means that we're making decisions amid "astounding levels of ignorance," as Lynn Goldman points out.[11]

"If you don't understand why something is harmful the best you can do is stay away from it," says Anastas, explaining our historical reliance on risk-avoidance. "We currently deal with chemical security through guns, guards, and gates rather than by redesigning materials. Protective measures against hazards can and will fail. And when they fail, risk goes to the maximum."[12]

❖ ❖ ❖

Green chemistry, if practiced thoroughly and honestly, could change all this. But much depends on that "if." John Warner, Terry Collins, Amy Cannon, James Hutchinson, Vicki Colvin, Paul Anastas, and other leading green chemistry proponents are quick to point out that green chemistry is a set of principles rather than a set of prescriptive or proscriptive standards. (Think green building's LEED standards or the criteria that qualify a product for the USDA organic label. Such a third-party certification program is *not* what green chemistry aspires to be.) Green chemistry aims to change a mind-set rather than to tweak, retrofit, or police. It aims to improve the entire nature of chemical synthesis rather than to regulate its products.

"Nothing is more important than design," says Anastas. "You can't do design by accident." To design materials that are inherently nontoxic, you must begin by asking the right sort of questions. For decades, by overlooking these questions about biological activity and ecological effects, synthetic chemistry has proceeded on assumptions that have sent us off, often far off, in the wrong direction where environmental health is concerned.

Green chemistry asks us to ask these questions from the very beginning of the molecular design process and at every step of chemical synthesis. Many of these questions have never been asked before as part of materials design. It is possible to argue that many of the manufactured chemicals now adrift in the atmosphere, the oceans, and our bodies were created before it was possible to answer any of these questions. Now that we have these tools it seems irresponsible not to use them to do what we can to prevent such problems from recurring.

Green chemistry would like these questions to be asked on the honor system. It's an idealistic strategy, but also a pragmatic one. Relying on a set of principles rather than certification standards avoids rules and labels, and offers carrots rather than sticks. Lack of mandatory hurdles will, in theory, encourage chemical industry participation. It's also useful politically, as it sets out a way to achieve environmental protection without new legislation or regulation. This strategy—if successful—also does away with the problem of lists of bans and their inevitable loopholes. Yet it seems clear to me that such a philosophical and entirely voluntary approach can only succeed if accompanied by serious reform in U.S. chemicals policy that will truly stop the current flow of hazardous chemicals and hold up some warning or directional signals to prevent greenwashing and false or inaccurate claims of safety.

Thus far, much existing environmental redesign and design of products and materials has been prompted, at least in part, by regulation or its specter—electronics are one example, cosmetics another. The European Union's REACH legislation may prove to be another. On the other hand, non-regulatory forces—growing consumer precaution and demand for alternatives to the current suite of hazardous ingredients—combined with a public skeptical of blanket assurances of product safety, may align to produce the results green chemists hope for.

To some extent, this is beginning to happen. Consumer demand is indeed spurring the development of new, environmentally benign synthetics and encouraging new product design that eliminates need for hazardous chemicals and promotes resource efficiency in materials and energy. Store shelves are now full of products proclaiming themselves resource-efficient and "free" of any number of potentially problematic synthetics. Yet verifying or assessing the worthiness of these claims remains difficult, and in some cases virtually impossible, thanks to the same system that's fostered the proliferation of problem chemicals. At the same time, new substances with even more unknown properties—nanomaterials—are rapidly proliferating. So I would argue that to achieve all that green chemistry aims to, particularly in this world of far-flung global supply chains, we also need an equally innovative and effective regulatory safety net.

Watching the response to current contaminant and climate change realities unfold over the past months, I believe we may be at something of a pivot point, where we seem to be rocking back and forth between the old world of problematic petrochemicals and halogenated hydrocarbons and a new universe of nontoxic, environmentally compatible synthetics derived from equally environmentally benign materials. The talk is tipped toward the environmentally benign and sustainable but the reality measurably far less so. As I read the news coming from the chemical industry and scientific community over the past year, I often pictured the Pushmi-Pullyu, the two-headed creature from *Dr. Doolittle* that always wanted to walk in opposite directions simultaneously. Major chemical manufacturers are formulating new lines of bio-based synthetics, developing alternatives to some long-used but ultimately hazardous compounds, and actively supporting green chemistry. At the same time the alliance between chemicals and petroleum—and the investment in petroleum—seems as tight as ever, as evidenced by recent business ventures linking major chemical companies with Middle Eastern oil producers.

To put this Pushmi-Pullyu dilemma firmly behind us in the United States will require significant new directions in policy. Central to this must be real transparency in chemical information that can protect proprietary commercial interests without sacrificing the vital public interest of true long-term environmental and human health protection. Based on our experience of how slowly and incompletely voluntary disclosure efforts produce results, it seems essential to establish more extensive mandatory programs to make information on the biological activity of chemicals fully available and up-to-date. Regulating on the basis of molecular design would go a long way toward establishing the basis of hazard and eliminating the secrecy that now obscures where that hazard may lie. And if environmental health protection is truly the goal it would also seem logical to put this information to work in a way that ensures that children in California, Canada, China, New York, and Belgium all receive the same—and maximum—health protections.

But gathering and disseminating information is only one step. We have reached a point where anthropogenically induced chemical imbalances in the world's environment exceed the scientific models now shaping public policy. We can wait longer until we reach greater and more costly crisis points or we can do what we've not done well before, and act now. Key to this will be continuing the collaboration that's just begun between environmental health scientists, synthetic chemists, and public health experts. Without this interaction it's unlikely that policy, principles, and practical solutions can come together swiftly enough.

When asked to assess the comparative impact of various environmental threats—climate change and global warming impacts, habitat loss and degradation, and pollution, none of which happen in isolation from each other—more than a handful of scientists have said to me, "It's hard to know which will be the straw that breaks the camel's back." When it comes to environmental chemical contamination, each individual exposure may be small, but their effects are now being felt everywhere at a time when ecological systems—from the deep ocean to the stratosphere—are responding to impacts for which they have limited innate defenses. And unlike other kinds of impacts to health and well-being, many of these contaminants are endocrine disruptors with effects that can span generations and that can occur before birth and alter health for a lifetime. The results of these chemical exposures are not hypothetical. They are with us and with our children now.

In economically difficult times, when thousands of jobs are being lost and covering basic living costs is difficult for many people, thinking about safer, greener materials—products that often carry a higher price tag—can seem like a luxury. It's hard to think about parts per billion or million of a tasteless, odorless, invisible substance that may or may not interact with your equally invisible genes and hormones when you're worried about paying the rent and feeding your children. But we can't afford not to make these changes—the consequences are too great. We need to find ways to make such products the norm rather than the exception. Green chemists caution against driving out the good in pursuit of the perfect and staunchly support any steps in their direction. Yet if we were to imagine the ideal, chemical hazard–free products would not be luxuries, nor would they require special diligence and education to find. They would simply be a given. Green chemistry alone cannot bring about these changes, but we cannot do this without green chemistry.

ACKNOWLEDGMENTS

There are many people without whose generosity and faith in me this book would not have been possible. Jonathan Cobb, my extraordinary editor, has shared his enthusiasm, encouragement, and expertise since I first began thinking about this project. My thanks to him are incalculable.

My great thanks to everyone at Island Press—including Todd Baldwin, Emily Davis, Jaime Jennings, Sharis Simonian, Brian Weese, George Abar, Krishna Roy, and Chuck Savitt—for their support and for providing a home for my work. The Overbrook Foundation and Oregon Literary Arts provided vital financial support for this book, for which I am deeply grateful. My thanks also to the Chemical Heritage Foundation for making it possible to use their library and attend the 2007 Gordon Cain Fellowship conference and to the Woods Hole Oceanographic Institution for opportunities provided by a science journalism fellowship there.

For inspiration, hospitality, and willingness to share information, there are more people than I can name here. Among those to whom special thanks are due are the entire science crew and Canadian Coast Guard Crew of the CCGS *Amundsen* for Leg 4B of the Circumpolar Flaw Lead System Study and the University of Manitoba Earth Systems Science Centre for inviting me on that amazing journey; to Pam Miller, Aluki

Brower, Viola Waghiyi, and Jesse Gologergen of Alaska Community Action on Toxics and the community of Savoonga for their welcome and generosity in sharing stories; to Tim Bates, Patricia Quinn, Eric Williams, Lynn Russell, and the rest of the ICEALOT crew for their patient explanations of atmospheric chemistry north of 66 degrees north; to Omana George and Sanjiv Pandita, their colleagues at ANROAV, and the Asia Monitor Resource Centre—my thanks and admiration. Among the others I would like to thank for their willingness to answer my questions, provide access to information and other resources, and for sharing enthusiasm for their work are Paul Anastas, Matthew Asplin, Dave Barber, Linda Birnbaum, Bruce Blumberg, Jeff Brook, Martina Buttler, Amy Cannon, Edward Chan, Theo Colborn, Terry Collins, Monica Danon-Schaffer, John Frazier, Andrea Gore, the Hagley Library and Archives, Tom Harner, Russ Hauser, Jerry Heindel, James Hutchinson, Dustin Isleifson, Liisa Jantunen, Captain Stéphane Julien, Barbara Karn, Dan Katz, Jane Kochersperger, Kristen Kulinowski, Dan Leitch, Robie Macdonald, Stacy Malkan, Alexandra McPherson, Andrew Maynard, Derek Muir, J. Peterson Myers, Retha Newbold, the Northeast Waste Management Officials Association, Karen O'Brien, the Othmer Library, Christopher Reddy, Jody Roberts, Mark Rossi, Frederick vom Saal, Ted Schettler, John Stegeman, Gary Stern, Shanna Swan, Christine Terada, Joel Tickner, Sarah Vogel, John Warner, and Michael Wilson. Again, there are far more people I would like to thank than there is room to name here.

Friends, colleagues, and editors who helped in all sorts of ways include Judith Alef, Jennifer Allen, Kevin Berger, Nils Bruzelius, David Campbell, John Carey, Peter Eisner, Susan Ewing, Douglas Fischer, Dave Gilson, Jim Hepworth, Cheryl Hogue, Andy Kerr, Pete Krsnak, Jonathan Leake, Gilly Lyons, Jason Mark, Ted Smith, John and Heather Sterling, Robert Stubblefield, Margot and George Thompson, and Katherine Wroth. Heartfelt thanks to my neighbors Susie Barnes, Hilary Bella, Theresa Koon, and Barb and Jordan Pahl for their help on the home front.

And as always, enormous thanks to my family—Alvin and Sari Grossman, Emily Grossman, Philip Zisman, and my nieces, Jane and Olivia—for encouraging boundless curiosity and for your love.

In *Green Chemistry: Theory and Practice*, Paul Anastas and John Warner outline what they call "the twelve principles of green chemistry." The principles listed here are as they appear at BeyondBenign.org with definitions adapted from the discussion in *Green Chemistry*.[1]

PRINCIPLES OF GREEN CHEMISTRY

1. Pollution Prevention: It is better to prevent waste than to treat or clean up waste after it is formed.

2. Atom Economy: Incorporate all atoms of starting materials into the final product to prevent waste and maximize resource efficiency.

3. Less Hazardous Synthesis: Use and design materials with little or no toxicity to human health and the environment.

4. Design Safer Chemicals

5. Safer Solvents and Auxiliaries: Minimize or eliminate the use of process chemicals, especially those that are hazardous.

6. Energy Efficiency

7. Renewable Feedstocks: Use renewable starting materials wherever possible.

8. Reduce Derivatives: Design synthetic processes that will maximize chemical and material efficiency and reduce hazardous waste and byproducts.

9. Catalysis: Design synthetic processes that maximize the efficiencies of catalytic reactions.

10. Design for Degradation: Design materials that will biodegrade into nontoxic products and not persist in the environment.

11. Real-Time Analysis: Monitor the synthetic process to detect and eliminate generation of hazardous waste and byproducts on an ongoing basis.

12. Accident Prevention: Choose materials and processes that will minimize the chances of accidents.

Paul Anastas has also devised what he calls a "molecular design pyramid," a series of questions to ask about materials, chemicals reactions, processes, and products that will help determine the probable environmental safety of a synthetic substance and process.[2] These are questions that have not typically been asked as new materials are being synthesized. These questions, like the twelve principles of green chemistry, are guides rather than prescriptive standards, but it should be evident that a material that is environmentally benign and without health hazards will not be persistent, bioaccumulative, or capable of disrupting or otherwise interfering with normally balanced function of cells and bodily systems (outside of specifically and intentionally targeted pharmaceutical applications).

MOLECULAR DESIGN PYRAMID QUESTIONS

- Is substance fat- or water-soluble? What's its potential to be persistent or to bioaccumulate?
- Is it volatile, explosive, flammable? What's its potential for atmospheric transport or deep lung penetration?
- What's its molecular weight?
- Can it partition to a gas?
- What's its electrical charge and how will this influence its physical and biochemical behavior?
- How will the molecule's shape, structure, and composition influence its bioavailability and mechanisms of its actions?
- Can it pass the blood-brain barrier? Can it penetrate the lungs, skin, or gastrointestinal tract? What's its potential for cellular absorption?
- What's its potential for genetic receptor binding?

NOTES

PROLOGUE

1. Author's interview with Paul Anastas, October 2007.
2. Paul T. Anastas and John C. Warner, *Green Chemistry: Theory and Practice* (New York: Oxford University Press, 1998), 8–9.
3. Anastas and Warner, *Green Chemistry*, 11.
4. Anastas and Warner, *Green Chemistry*, 13.
5. Anastas and Warner, *Green Chemistry*, 11.
6. Author's interview with John Warner, May 2007.
7. John C. Warner, "Guest Editorial: Asking the Right Questions,"*Green Chemistry* 6, no. 1 (2004): 27–28.
8. The EPA's Green Chemistry and Design for the Environment programs are now under this umbrella.

CHAPTER 1: THERE'S SOMETHING IN THE AIR

1. U.S. Environmental Protection Agency, "Contaminants in Great Lakes Sport Fish Fillets," www.epa.gov/glindicators/fishtoxics/sportfishb.html.
2. Elaine MacDonald and Sarah Rang, *Exposing Canada's Chemical Valley: An Investigation of Cumulative Air Pollution Emissions in Sarnia, Ontario Area*, Toronto: (Ecojustice, 2007); Martin Mittelstadt, "Sarnia's Emissions Affecting Health, Study Says," *Toronto Globe & Mail*, October 4, 2007; Karen Y, Fung, Isaac N. Luginaah, and Kevin M. Gorcy, "Impact of Air Pollution on Hospital

Admissions in Southwestern Ontario, Canada: Generating Hypotheses in Sentinel High-Exposure Places," *Environmental Health* 6, no. 18 (July 2007).

3. MacDonald and Rang, "Exposing Canada's Chemical Valley."

4. Kellyn Betts, "Unwelcome Guest: PBDES in Indoor Dust," *Environmental Health Perspectives* 116, no. 5 (2008): A202–8.

5. Marina Fernández, Maria Bianchi, Victoria Lux-Lantos, and Carlos Libertun, "Neonatal Exposure to Bisphenol A Alters Reproductive Parameters and Gonadotropin Releasing Hormone Signaling in Female Rats," *Environmental Health Perspectives* 117, no. 5 (2009): 757–62. See also Julia R. Barrett, "Trumped Treatment? BPA Blocks Effects of Breast Cancer Chemotherapy Drugs," *Environmental Health Perspectives* 117, no. 2.

6. See Centers for Disease Control NHANES reports.

7. Shanna H. Swan, personal communication with author, March 2007.

8. Terrence J. Collins and Chip Walter, "Little Green Molecules," *Scientific American*, March 2006, 84.

9. John Warner, personal communication with author, May 2007.

10. Christopher M. Reddy, John J. Stegeman, and Mark E. Hahn, "Organic Pollutants: Presence and Effects in Humans and Marine Animals," in *Oceans and Human Health*, ed. P. J. Walsh, S. L. Smith, H. Solo-Gabriele, and W. H. Gerwick (Boston: Elsevier, 2008), 121–44.

11. John Stegeman, in discussion with the author, September 2008.

12. Michael P. Wilson with Daniel A. Chia and Bryan C. Ehlers, *Green Chemistry in California: A Framework for Leadership in Chemicals Policy and Innovation* (Berkeley: University of California Press, 2006).

13. Wilson, Chia, and Ehlers, *Green Chemistry in California*. See also U.S. EPA High Production Volume Challenge Program.

14. Ken Geiser, *Materials Matter: Toward a Sustainable Materials Policy* (Cambridge, Mass.: MIT Press, 2001), 3.

15. Comments by Derek Muir made at the AAAS 2008 conference.

16. Paul T. Anastas and John C. Warner, *Green Chemistry: Theory and Practice* (New York: Oxford University Press, 1998), 9.

17. The "Twelve Principles of Green Chemistry" are listed in the appendix to this volume (see page 203).

18. Paul J. Crutzen, "Geology of Mankind," *Nature* 415, no. 3 (2002): 23.

CHAPTER 2: SWIMMERS, HOPPERS, AND FLIERS

This characterization of "swimmers, hoppers, and flyers" is taken from Dr. Frank Wania's research, as described in Todd Gouin and Frank Wania, "Time Trends of Arctic Contamination in Relation to Emission History and Chemical Persistence and Partitioning Properties," *Environmental Science and Technology* 41, no. 17 (2007): 5986–97, and other papers.

1. Arctic Monitoring and Assessment Programme (AMAP) and Arctic Council Action Plan to Eliminate Pollution of the Arctic (ACAP), "Fact Sheet: Brominated Flame Retardants in the Arctic," January 2005, www.amap.no/.

2. Karla Pozo, Tom Harner, Frank Wania, Derek C. G. Muirm Kevin C. Jones, and Leonard A. Barrie, "Toward a Global Network for Persistent Organic Pollutants in Air: Results from the GAPS Study," *Environmental Science & Technology* 40 (2006): 4867–73.

3. This study is the Western Airborne Contaminants Assessment Project, designed and implemented by the National Park Service in January 2008.

4. Author's interview with Eric Dewailly, March 2008.

5. See the Stockholm Convention on Persistent Organic Pollutants, http://chm .pops.int/Convention/tabid/54/language/enP-US/Default.aspx.

6. Stockholm Convention on Persistent Organic Pollutants, "Governments Unite to Step-Up Reduction on Global DDT Reliance and Add Nine New Chemicals under International Treaty," press release, May 9, 2009, http://chm.pops.int/ Convention/Pressrelease/COP4Geneva8May2009/tabid/542/language/en-US/Default.aspx.

7. Gouin and Wania, "Time Trends of Arctic Contamination," 5986–92. R. W. Macdonald, D. Mackay, Y.-F. Li, and B. Hickie, "How Will Global Climate Change Affect Risks from Long-Range Transport of Persistent Organic Pollutants?" *Human and Ecological Risk Assessment* 9, no. 3 (2003): 644–45.

8. Torsten Meyer and Frank Wania, "What Environmental Fate Processes Have the Strongest Influence on a Completely Persistent Organic Chemical's Accumulation in the Arctic?" *Atmospheric Environment* 41 (2007): 2757–67. Quotation from page 2763.

9. Author's interview with Derek Muir, February 2008.

10. Heidi N. Geisz, Rebecca M. Dickhut, Michele A. Cochran, William R. Fraser, and Hugh W. Ducklow, "Melting Glaciers: A Probable Source of DDT to the Antarctic Marine Ecosystem," *Environmental Science & Technology* 42 (2008): 3958–62, http://pubs.acs.org/cgi-bin/article.cgi/esthag/2008/42/i11/pdf/es 702919n.pdf?isMac=23773.

11. Doug Struck, "Dust Storms Overseas Carry Contaminants to U.S.," *Washington Post,* February 6, 2008.

12. Lori Styles, University Communications, "UA Scientist Leads U.N. Team Drafting Plan For Sand, Dust Storm Warning System," *UA News,* November 20, 2007, http://uanews.org/node/17041.

13. United States National Snow and Ice Data Center, "Arctic Sea Ice News

& Analysis," University of Colorado, Boulder, http://nsidc.org/arcticseaice
news/index.html.

14. Tatiana Savinova, Vladimir Savinov, Lyudmila Stephanova, Sergey Kotelevtsev,
    Geir Wing Gabrielsen, and Janneche Utne Skaare, "Biological Effects of POPs
    on Svalbard Glaucous Gulls," Norwegian Ministry of the Environment, www
    .npolar.no/transeff/Effects/Glaucous_Gull/Gull-Akvaplan.htm. See also http://
    npweb.npolar.no/english/articles/1207829685.63.

CHAPTER 3: LABORATORY CURIOSITIES AND CHEMICAL UNKNOWNS

1. Centers for Disease Control and Prevention, "Childhood Overweight and Obesity," February 10, 2009, www.cdc.gov/nccdphp/dnpa/obesity/childhood/.

2. "Cost Estimates as a Guide to Research," proposed talk to be delivered before
   Louisville Section National Association of Cost Accountants, February 15,
   1955. Hagley Museum and Library Collection.

3. Research progress report for Feb. 1935 P-16 E. I. DuPont de Nemours & Co.,
   Wilmington, Delaware. Chemical Department, Experimental Station, Hagley
   Museum and Library. See also June 27, 1935, DuPont Cellophane Company
   Inc., memo from O. F. Benz, D. S. to Dr. W. H. Charch, P-19 Pioneering Re-
   search Division, Subject: Visking Corporation—Sausage Casing, Hagley Mu-
   seum and Library.

4. January 21, 1935. Dr. H. E. Eastlack, Attention: Mr. P. M. Clark, DuPont Archives, Hagley.

5. See Gerald Markowitz and David Rosner, *Deceit and Denial: The Deadly Politics
   of Industrial Polution* (Berkeley: University of California Press, 2002).

6. C. L. Burdick, Development Department, Pioneering Research Division,
   DuPont de Nemours & Company, "Synthetic Plastics: Industrial Value of the
   Vinyl Derivatives," *Chemical Trade Journal*, August 14, 1936, Hagley Museum
   and Library.

7. Daniel Yergin, *The Prize: The Epic Quest for Oil, Money, and Power* (New York:
   Simon & Schuster, 1991), 259.

8. Christopher Reddy, personal communication with author, September 2007

9. Yergin, *The Prize*, 15.

10. Rachel Carson, *Silent Spring* (Boston: Houghton Mifflin, 1994), 7.

11. Carson, *Silent Spring*, 187.

12. Carson, *Silent Spring*, 30.

13. Theo Colborn, Dianne Dumanoski, and John Peterson Myers, *Our Stolen Fu-*

ture: Are We Threatening Our Fertility, Intelligence, and Survival? A Scientific Detective Story (New York: Dutton, 1996). See especially chapter 1.

14. Linda Birnbaum, Dioxin 2007, Tokyo, September 2007.

15. Author's interview with Linda S. Birnbaum, September 2007.

16. Peter C. Juliano, General Electric Company, "1985—Science and Technology of Polymer Blends," accessed at Chemical Heritage Foundation, Othmer Library.

17. AAAS February 16, 2008, presentation by Nat Scholz and John Incardona, fisheries biologies with the National Oceanic and Atmospheric Administration (NOAA) on effects of pesticides on salmon.

CHAPTER 4: THE POLYCARBONATE PROBLEM

1. National Institute of Environmental Health Sciences, "Since You Asked— Bisphenol A: Questions and Answers about the National Toxicology Program's Evaluation of Bisphenol A," www.niehs.nih.gov/news/media/questions/sya-bpa.cfm.

2. Elvira Greiner, Thomas Kaelin, and Kazuaki Nakamura, "Bisphenol A" (SRI Consulting, November 2007), www.sriconsulting.com/CEH/Public/Reports/619.5000/.

3. American Chemistry Council, "Bisphenol-A Website." www.bisphenol-a.org.

4. In 2007, General Electric sold its plastics division to the Saudi Arabian company SABIC (Saudi Basic Industries Corporation), which makes chemicals, plastics, fertilizers, and metals.

5. American Chemistry Council, "About Bisphenol-A," www.bisphenol-a.org/about/index.html.

6. F. S. vom Saal, B. T. Akingbemi, S. M. Belcher, L. S. Birnbaum, D. A. Crain, M. Eriksen, F. Farabollini, et al., "Chapel Hill Bisphenol A Expert Panel Consensus Statement: Integration of Mechanisms, Effects in Animals, and Potential to Impact Human Health at Current Levels of Exposure," *Reproductive Toxicology* 24, no. 2 (2007): 131–38.

7. Julia A. Taylor, Wade. V. Welshons, and Frederick S. vom Saal, "No Effect of Route of Exposure (Oral; Subcutaneous Injection) on Plasma Bisphenol A throughout 24 Hours after Administration in Neonatal Female Mice," *Reproductive Toxicology* 25, no. 2 (2007): 169–76.

8. Antonia M. Calafat, Zsuzsanna Kuklenyik, John A. Reidy, Samuel P. Caudill, John Ekong, and Larry L. Needham, "Urinary Concentrations of Bisphenol A and 4-Nonylphenol in a Human Reference Population," *Environmental Health Perspectives*, 113, no. 4 (2005): 391–95.

9. Environmental Working Group, "A Survey of Bisphenol A in U.S. Canned Foods," March 5, 2007, www.ewg.org/reports/bisphenola.

10. American Chemistry Council, "Epoxy Resin Can Coatings and Bisphenol A Safety Information." www.bisphenol-a.org/human/epoxycan.html.

11. Nancy K. Wilson, Jane C. Chuang, Christopher Lyu, Ronald Menton, and Marsha K. Morgan, "Aggregate Exposures of Nine Preschool Children to Persistent Organic Pollutants at Day Care and at Home," *Journal of Exposure Analysis and Environmental Epidemiology* 13 (2003): 187–202. See also Nancy K. Wilson, Jane C. Chuang, Marsha K. Morgan, R. A. Lordo, and L. S. Sheldon, "An Observation Study of the Potential Exposures of Preschool Children to Pentachlorophenol, Bisphenol-A, and Nonylphenol at Home and Daycare," *Environmental Research* 103, no. 1 (2006): 9–20.

12. Martin Mittelstaedt, "Tests Find Bisphenol A in Majority of Soft Drinks," *Globe & Mail,* March 5, 2009, www.theglobeandmail.com/servlet/story/LAC.20090305.BPA05/TPStory.

13. Jenny L. Carwile, Henry T. Luu, Laura S. Bassett, Daniel A. Driscoll, Caterina Yuan, Jennifer Y. Chang, Xiaoyun Ye, Antonia M. Calafat, and Karin B. Michels, "Use of Polycarbonate Bottles and Urinary Bisphenol A Concentrations," *Environmental Health Perspectives* doi:10.1289/ehp.0900604, www.ehponline.org/docs/2009/0900604/abstract.pdf, accessed May 12, 2009.

14. Hugh S. Taylor, personal communication with author, March 2007.

15. See E. C. Dodds and Wilfrid Lawson, "Synthetic Oestrogenic Agents without the Phenanthrene Nucleus," *Nature*, June 13, 1936, 996; J. W. Cook and E. C. Dodds, "Sex Hormones and Cancer-Producing Compounds," *Nature*, February 11, 1933, 205–6; J. W. Cook, E. C. Dodds, and C. L. Hewett, "A Synthetic Oetrus-Exciting Compound," *Nature*, January 14, 1933, 56–57; and J. W. Cook, C. Hewett, and I. Hieger, "Coal Tar Constituents and Cancer," *Nature*, December 17, 1932, 926–27.

16. Transcript of an Interview with Daniel W. Fox conducted by Leonard W. Fine and George Wise at Pittsfield, Mass., on August 14, 1986, accessed at Chemical Heritage Foundation, Othmer Library.

17. Rachel Carson, *Silent Spring* (Boston: Houghton Mifflin, 1994), 204.

18. Transcript of an Interview with Daniel W. Fox conducted by Leonard W. Fine and George Wise at Pittsfield, Mass., on August 14, 1986, accessed at Chemical Heritage Foundation, Othmer Library.

19. Daniel W. Fox—Recent Developments in Engineering Plastics Polymer Blends DWF [7-2] Blends—1983 (2 of 2), accessed at Chemical Heritage Foundation, Othmer Library.

20. "56.924 Polycarbonate Resins," *Federal Register* 42, no. 50, March 15, 1977.

21. All toxicity information from the Agency for Toxic Substances and Disease Registry's (ATSDR's) ToxFAQs, www.atsdr.cdc.gov/toxfaq.html.

22. Memo Report: "Use of Butanediol-(bis-glycidylether) as a Hydrolytic Stabilizer for Lexan Resin," February 15, 1978, General Electric, Lexan Department, Mt. Vernon, Indiana, accessed at Chemical Heritage Foundation, Othmer Library

23. American Chemistry Council, "FAQs: The Safety of Baby Bottles, Nalgene Sports Bottles, and Food Containers Made with Polycarbonate Plastic," www .plasticsinfo.org/s_plasticsinfo/sec_level2_faq.asp?CID=704&DID=2838.

24. U.S. Environmental Protection Agency, "Bisphenol A," January 10, 2008. www.epa.gov/iris/subst/0356.htm.

25. Sarah Vogel, "Battles over Bisphenol A," DefendingScience.org, April 16, 2008, www.defendingscience.org/case_studies/Battles-Over-Bisphenol-A.cfm.

26. Theo Colborn, Dianne Dumanoski, and John Peterson Myers, *Our Stolen Future: Are We Threatening Our Fertility, Intelligence, and Survival? A Scientific Detective Story* (New York: Dutton, 1996). See especially chapter 8, excerpts available at www.ourstolenfuture.org/Basics/chapter_excerpts/8herethere.htm.

27. Author's interview with Patricia Hunt, February 2007.

28. Elizabeth W. LaPensee, Traci R. Tuttle, Sejal R. Fox, and Nira Ben-Jonathan, "Bisphenol A at Low Nanomolar Doses Confers Chemoresistance in Estrogen-Receptor-Alpha-Positive and -Negative Breast Cancer Cells," *Environmental Health Perspectives* 117, no. 2 (2009): 175–80. Laura N. Vandenberg, Russ Hauser, Michele Marcus, Nocolas Olea, and Wade V. Welshons. "Human Exposure to Bisphenol A (BPA)," *Reproductive Toxicology* 24, no. 2 (2007): 139–77. Csaba Leranth, Tibor Hajszan, Klara Szigeti-Buck, Jeremy Bober, and Niel J. MacLusky. "Bisphenol A Prevents the Synaptogenic Response to Estradiol in Hippocampus and Prefrontal Cortex of Ovariectomized Nonhuman Primates," *Proceedings of the National Academy of Sciences* 105, no. 37 (2008): 14187–91.

29. Frederick S. vom Saal, personal communication with author, March 2007.

30. Andrea Gore, personal communication with author, March 2007.

31. General Electric company memos 1984, accessed at the Chemical Heritage Foundation, Othmer Library.

32. Kembra L. Howdeshell, Paul H. Peterman, Barbara M. Judy, Julia A. Taylor, Carl E. Orazio, Rachel L. Ruhlen, Frederick S. Vom Saal, and Wade V. Welshons, "Bisphenol A Is Released from Used Polycarbonate Animal Cages into Water," *Environmental Health Perspectives* 111, no. 9 (2003): 1180–87.

33. Martha Susiarjo, Terry J. Hassold, Edward Freeman, and Patricia A. Hunt, "Bisphenol A Exposure in Utero Disrupts Early Oogenesis in the Mouse,"

PLoS Genetics 3, no. 1 (2007): e5, www.plosgenetics.org/article/info:doi/10
.1371/journal.pgen.0030005.

34. Caroline C. Smith and Hugh S. Taylor, "Xenoestrogen Exposure Imprints Expression of Genes (Hoxa10) Required for Normal Uterine Development," *The FASEB Journal* 21 (2007): 239–46.

35. Bisphenol A affects the male reproductive hormone systems as well as the female's. There has been extensive research into its impacts on testosterone, prostate, and other male body systems.

36. Hugh S. Taylor, personal communication with author, March 2007.

37. Patricia A. Hunt, personal communication with author, March 2007.

38. F. S. vom Saal, B. T. Akingbemi, S. M. Belcher, L. S. Birnbaum, D. A. Crain, M. Eriksen, F. Farabollini, et al., "Chapel Hill Bisphenol A Expert Panel Consensus Statement: Integration of Mechanisms, Effects in Animals and Potential to Impact Human Health at Current Levels of Exposure," *Reproductive Toxicology* 24, no. 2 (2007): 131–38.

39. Patricia A. Hunt, personal communication with author, March 2007.

40. Retha R. Newbold, "Prenatal Exposure to Diethylstilbestrol (DES)," *Fertility and Sterility* 89, supp. 1 (2008): e55–e56, www.prhe.ucsf.edu/prhe/prhe_articles/14.FertSter2008.Sup1.Newbold.pdf.

41. A. P. Raun and R. L. Preston, "History of Diethylstilbestrol Use in Cattle." Unplublished paper, American Society of Animal Science, 2002 www.asas.org/Bios/Raunhist.pdf.

42. Retha R. Newbold, personal communication with author, February 2007, and comments made at the AAAS 2007 conference.

43. For a helpful explanation of epigenetics see Joanna Downer, "Backgrounder: Epigenetics and Imprinted Genes," Johns Hopkins Medicine, November 15, 2002, www.hopkinsmedicine.org/press/2002/november/epigenetics.htm.

44. Comments by John Peterson Myers made at the AAAS 2007 conference.

45. Philippe Grandjean, David Bellinger, Åke Bergman, Sylvaine Cordier, George Davey-Smith, Brenda Eskenazi, David Gee, et al., "The Faroes Statement: Human Health Effects of Developmental Exposure to Environmental Toxicants," International Conference on Fetal Programming and Environmental Toxicity, May 20–24, 2007, www.pptox.dk/Consensus/tabid/72/Default.aspx.

46. Comments by Newbold and Blumberg made at the 2007 AAAS Conference.

47. Organotins are a subset of compounds known as organometallics (substances made up of metals and hydrocarbons). Organometallics include methyl mercury and tetraethyl lead, both known for their biological toxicity.

48. The information bulletin is Cornell University's Extension Toxicology Network (ETOXNET), http://pmep.cce.cornell.edu/profiles/extoxnet/pyrethrins-ziram/tributyltin-ext.html.

49. These effects have resulted in an international agreement that discontinues tributyltin's use in anti-fouling paints used on ships. A similar U.S. law, the Organotin Antifouling Paint Control Act, was passed in 1988 but as of this writing the EPA continues to assess other applications of tributyltin.

50. Author's interview with Bruce Blumberg, February 2007.

51. F. S. vom Saal, J. R. Kirkpatrick, and B. L. Coe, "Environmental Estrogens, Endocrine Disruption, and Obesity," in *Obesity: Epidemiology, Pathophysiology, and Prevention*, ed. Debasis Bagchi and Harry G. Preuss (Boca Raton, Fla.: CRC Press, 2006), 33–41.

52. Richard W. Stalhut, Edward van Wijngaarden, Timothy D. Dye, Stephen Cook, and Shanna H. Swan, "Concentrations of Urinary Phthalate Metabolites Are Associated with Increased Waist Circumference and Insulin Resistance in Adult U.S. Males," *Environmental Health Perspectives* 115, no. 6 (2007): 876–82.

53. Joseph L. Jacobson and Sandra W. Jacobson, "Intellectual Impairment in Children Exposed to Polychlorinated Biphenyls in Utero," *New England Journal of Medicine* 335, no. 11 (1996): 783–89; See also Paul W. Stewart, Edward Lonky, Jacqueline Reihman, James Pagano, Brooks B. Gump, and Thomas Darvill, "The Relationship between Prenatal PCB Exposure and Intelligence (IQ) in 9-Year-Old Children," *Environmental Health Perspectives* 116, no. 10 (2008): 1416–22.

54. Bernard Weiss, "Neurobiology and Behavior," University of Rochester, www2.envmed.rochester.edu/envmed/tox/faculty/weiss.html.

55. Bernard Weiss, "Can Endocrine Disruptors Influence Neuroplasticity in the Aging Brain?" *NeuroToxicology* 28, no. 5 (2007): 938–50.

56. Weiss, "Endocrine Disruptors."

57. Draft NTP Brief on Bisphenol A [CAS No.80-05-7], April 14, 2008, National Toxicology Program, National Institute of Environmental Health Sciences, National Institutes of Health, Department of Health and Human Services. Also see National Institute of Environmental Health Sciences, "NTP Finalized Report on Bisphenol A," press release, September 3, 2008, www.niehs.nih.gov/news/releases/2008/bisphenol-a.cfm.

58. vom Saal et al., "Chapel Hill Bisphenol A Expert Panel."

59. In April 2008, Wal-Mart announced it would discontinue the sale of baby bottles, pacifiers, toddlers' sippy cups, or water bottles made with bisphenol A in its Canadian stores; U.S. Wal-Mart stores would follow suit starting in early

2009. Other big retailers, including Toys "R" Us, the Mountain Equipment Co-Op (Canada's largest sports retailer), and the CVS pharmacy chain have developed similar policies; half a dozen manufacturers of baby bottles, including Gerber and Playtex, have since discontinued their bisphenol A products.

60. "Ottawa to Ban Baby Bottles Made with Bisphenol A," CBC News, April 18, 2008.

61. Eastman, "New Eastman Tritan Copolyester," www.eastman.com/Brands/ Tritan/Introduction/Introduction.htm.

62. U.S. Food and Drug Administration, "Bisphenol A (BPA)," www.fda.gov/ oc/opacom/hottopics/bpa.html.

63. American Chemistry Council, "Are the Myths about Polycarbonate Bottles True? New Information Supports the Safe Use of Polycarbonate Bottles," February 5, 2008, www.bisphenol-a.org/whatsNew/20080205.html.

64. American Chemistry Council, "Are the Myths about Polycarbonate Bottles True?" See the Bisphenol A website at www.bisphenol-a.org/whatsNew/ 20080205.html, accessed April 10, 2009.

65. American Chemistry Council, "Pthalates Information Center," www .phthalates.org/didyouknow/myth.asp.

66. Jennifer Muir, "Industry Fights Effort to Ban Chemical in Baby Products," *Orange County Register*, August 8, 2008.

67. Lyndsey Layton, "Studies on Chemical in Plastics Questioned," *Washington Post*, April 27, 2008.

68. U.S. Environmental Protection Agency, "Risk Assessment for Toxic Air Pollutants: A Citizen's Guide," originally published as EPA 450/3-90-024, March 1991, www.epa.gov/ttn/atw/3_90_024.html.

69. Joel Tickner, personal communication with author, June 2008.

70. For more information about this group, see http://stats.org/.

71. Trevor Butterworth, "*Washington Post* Skews Story on Chemical Obesity Risk," STATS, March 12, 2007, http://stats.org/stories/2007/washington_obesity_ mar12_07.htm.

72. George Gray and Joshua Cohen, "Weight of the Evidence Evaluation of Low-Dose Reproductive and Developmental Effects of Bisphenol A," *Risk in Perspective* 12, no. 3 (2004): 1–4, www.hcra.harvard.edu/rip/risk_in_persp_August 2004.pdf.

73. For a list of the reviewed studies, see www.gradientcorp.com/publications/ scientificpapers.php.

74. For Meghan Reilly's research report, see www.cga.ct.gov/2008/rpt/2008-

R-0249.htm. For further information, see www.senate.mn/committees/2007-2008/health/update.htm.

75. Samantha Young, "California Lawmakers Weigh Ban on Chemical Found in Baby Bottles, although Danger Is in Dispute," Associated Press, August 10, 2008. For Julie F. Goodman's comments on behalf of the American Petroleum Institute, see http://yosemite.epa.gov/sab/sabproduct.nsf/519F483722AAA 80485257494006205F1/$File/Goodman_CASAC+SOx+Public+Comments+ for+July+30-31+2008+Meeting.pdf. I also discovered that STATS is listed among the bisphenol A information recommended by the Juvenile Products Manufacturing Association website and STATS staff are authors of the JPMA statement defending bisphenol A safety.

76. For more information on STATS, see www.stats.org/about.htm. I came by this information via Guidestar and SourceWatch.

77. For more information on the Endocrine Disruption Exchange (TEDX), see www.endocrinedisruption.com/home.php.

78. John Tierney, "Ten Things to Scratch from Your Worry List," *New York Times*, science section, July 29, 2008. NB: The print edition carried a teaser-headline that included the word "myth." It is not in the web edition.

CHAPTER 5: PLASTICIZERS: HEALTH RISKS OR FIFTY YEARS OF DENIAL OF DATA?

1. Marla Cone, "Scientists Find 'Baffling' Link between Autism and Vinyl Flooring," *Environmental Health News*, March 31, 2009, www.environmentalhealth news.org/ehs/news/autism-and-vinyl-flooring. See also Malin Larssona, Bernard Weiss, Staffan Janson, Jan Sundell, and Carl-Gustav Bornehag, "Associations between Indoor Environmental Factors and Parental-Reported Autistic Spectrum Disorders in Children 6–8 Years of Age," *NeuroToxicology*, forthcoming.

2. For the final text of HR 4040, section 108, see http://thomas.loc.gov/cgi-bin/bdquery/z?d110:h.r.04040: and follow links to text of bill. The bills are HR 4040 and S 2663, laws that also ban all but the merest trace of lead from products intended for children under twelve years old. The six phthalate formulations are diethylhexyl phthalate (DEHP also referred to as di-2-ethylhexyl phthalate), dibutyl phthalate (DBP, sometimes also referred to as di-n-butyl phthalate), benzyl butyl phthalate (BBP), diisononyl phthalate (DINP), diisodecyl phthalate (DIDP), and di-n-octyl phthalate (DnOP).

3. Canada has barred two of the most widely used phthalates, diethylhexyl

phthalate (DEHP) and diiosononyl phthalate (DINP), both of which go into PVC, from infants' and children's products since 1998.

4. Benjamin C. Blount, Manori J. Silva, Samuel P. Caudill, Larry L. Needham, Jim L. Pirkle, Eric J. Sampson, George W. Lucier, et al., "Levels of Seven Urinary Phthalate Metabolites in a Human Population," *Environmental Health Perspectives* 108, no. 10 (2000): 979–82.

5. Author's interview with Shanna Swan, March 2007.

6. UK Food Standards Agency, "Food Surveillance Information Sheet," no. 60, May 1995, http://archive.food.gov.uk/maff/archive/food/infsheet/1995/no60/60phthal.htm.

7. Sheela Sathyanarayana, Catherine J. Karr, Paula Lozano, Elizabeth Brown, Antonia M. Calafat, Fan Liu, and Shanna H. Swan, "Baby Care Products: Possible Sources of Infant Phthalate Exposure," *Pediatrics* 121, no. 2 (2008): e260–e268.

8. Theo Colborn, Dianne Dumanoski, and John Peterson Myers, *Our Stolen Future: Are We Threatening Our Fertility, Intelligence, and Survival? A Scientific Detective Story* (New York: Dutton, 1996). See especially "Hypospadias in the U.S.," excerpts available at www.ourstolenfuture.org/NEWSCIENCE/reproduction/hypospadias.htm.

9. John D. Meeker, Antonia M. Calafat, and Russ Hauser, "Di(2-ethylhexyl) Phthalate Metabolites May Alter Thyroid Hormone Levels in Men," *Environmental Health Perspectives* 115, no. 7 (2007): 1029–34.

10. Jennifer J. Adibi, Russ Hauser, Paige L. Williams, Robin M. Whyatt, Antonia M. Calafat, Heather Nelson, Robert Herrick, and Shanna H. Swan, "Maternal Urinary Metabolites of Di(2-Ethylhexyl) Phthalate in Relation to the Timing of Labor in a U.S. Multicenter Pregnancy Cohort Study," *American Journal of Epidemiology*, forthcoming.

11. Manori J. Silva, John A. Reidy, James L. Preau Jr., Larry L. Needham, and Antonia M. Calafat, "Oxdative Metabolites of Diisononyl Pthalate as Biomarkers for Human Exposure Assessment," *Environmental Health Perspectives* 114, no. 8 (2006): 1158–61.

12. Paul Foster, personal communication with the author, March 2007.

13. Peter Infante, Stephen E. Petty, David H. Groth, Gerald Markowitz, and David Rosner, "Vinyl Chloride Propellant in Hair Spray and Angiosarcoma of the Liver among Hairdressers and Barbers: Case Reports," *International Journal of Occupational and Environmental Health*, 15, no. 1 (2009): 36–42.

14. Environment California, "Phthalates Overview," www.environmentcalifornia.org/environmental-health/stop-toxic-toys/phthalates-overview.

15. Meg Kissinger and Susanne Rust, "U.S. Lawmakers Move to Ban BPA from Food, Beverage Containers," *Milwaukee Journal Sentinel*, March 13, 2009.

16. For the American Chemistry Council's response to NPR's piece on the phthalate ban, see "ACC Responds," www.americanchemistry.com/s%5Fphthalate/sec.asp?CID=2084&DID=8774. For the original NPR article, see Jon Hamilton, "Public Concern, Not Science, Prompts Plastics Ban," National Public Radio, April 1, 2009, www.npr.org/templates/story/story.php?storyId=102567295.

17. National Toxicology Program, "Chemical Information Profile for Diethyl Phthalate CAS No.84-66-2, Supporting Nomination for Toxicological Evaluation," November 2006. Prepared for National Toxicology Program.

18. Jun Sekizawa, Stuart Dobson, and Ralph J. Touch III, "Concise International Chemical Document 52: Diethyl Phthalate," www.inchem.org/documents/cicads/cicads/cicad52.htm.

19. Agency for Toxic Substances and Disease Registry, "ToxFAQs for Diethyl Phthalate," www.atsdr.cdc.gov/tfacts73.html.

20. Comments by Paul Foster made during his presentation at Chemical Heritage Foundation, Gordon Cain Conference, March 2007.

21. Comments by Paul Foster made during his presentation at Chemical Heritage Foundation, Gordon Cain Conference, March 2007.

22. American Chemistry Council, "The Body of Scientific Evidence on Phthalates," press teleconference by Chris Bryant, managing director, chemical products and technology division, August 18, 2008.

23. American Chemistry Council, "Phthalates Information Center," http://www.americanchemistry.com/s_phthalate/index.asp.

24. G. Wildbrett, "Diffusion of Phthalate Acid Esters from PVC Milk Tubing," *Environmental Health Perspectives* 3 (1973): 29–35.

25. Frederick C. Gross and Joe A. Colony, "The Ubiquitous Nature and Objectionable Characteristics of Phthalate Esters in Aerospace Technology," *Environmental Health Perspectives* 3 (1973): 37–48.

26. W. J. Olewinski, G. Rapier, T. K. Slawecki, and H. Warner, "Investigation of Toxic Properties of Materials Used in Space Vehicles, Technical Documentary Report No. AMRL-TDR-63-99," December 1963, Biomedical Laboratory, Aerospace Medical Division, Air Force Systems Command, Wright-Patterson Air Force Base, Ohio, Prepared Under Contract No. AF-33(657)-8029, General Electric Company, Missile and Space Division, Philadelphia, PA.

27. Paul R. Mahaffy, David Beaty, Mark Anderson, Glenn Aveni, Jeff Bada, Simon Clemett, David Des Marais, et al., "Science Priorities Related to the Organic

Contamination of Martian Landers," unpublished white paper, November 2004, Mars Exploration Program Analysis Group (MEPAG), http://mepag.jpl.nasa.gov/reports/index.html.

28. Dean Finney, Phthalate Esters Panel of the American Chemistry Council teleconference, August 2008.

29. Rebecca Goldin, "Toy Tantrums: The Debate over the Safety of Phthalates," STATS, January 30, 2006, http://stats.org/stories/2008/the_risks_phthalates_mar24_08.html. See also American Chemistry Council, "Media Alert: Consumer Products that Do Not Contain Phthalates," July 14, 2008, www.americanchemistry.com/s_phthalate/sec.asp?CID=2054&DID=8630.

30. Ted Schettler, personal communication with author, August 2008. Dr. Ted Schettler, MD, is science director of the nonprofit Science Environmental Health Network.

31. Meeker et al., "Di(2-ethylhexyl) Phthalate Metabolites."

32. Jennifer Weuve, Brisa N. Sánchez, Antonia M. Calafat, Ted Schettler, Ronald A. Green, Howard Hu, and Russ Hauser, "Exposure to Phthalates in Neonatal Intensive Care Unit Infants: Urinary Concentrations of Monoesters and Oxidative Metabolites," *Environmental Health Perspectives* 114, no. 9 (2006): 1424–31. See also Tom Deutschle, Rudolf Reiter, Werner Butte, Berger Heinzow, Tilman Keck, and Herbert Riechelmann, "A Controlled Challenge Study on Di(2-ethylhexyl) Phthalate (DEHP) in House Dust and the Immune Response in Human Nasal Mucosa of Allergic Subjects," *Environmental Health Perspectives* 116, no. 11 (2008): 1487–93. See also Rie Yanagisawa, Hirohisa Takano, Kenichiro Inoue, Eiko Koike, Kaori Sadakane, and Takamichi Ichinose, "Effects of Maternal Exposure to Di-(2-ethylhexyl) Phthalate during Fetal and/or Neonatal Periods on Atopic Dermatitis in Male Offspring," *Environmental Health Perspectives* 116, no. 9 (2008): 1136–41.

33. DPB Information Centre, "DBP: A Specialty Plasticiser," www.dbp-facts.com.

34. Bette Hileman, "Panel Ranks Risks of Common Phthalate: Additional Research Underscores Concerns about DEHP That Were First Expressed in 2000 Report," *Chemical & Engineering News* 83, no. 46 (2005): 32–36.

35. Center for the Evaluation of Risks to Human Reproduction, National Toxicology Program, "NTP Brief on the Potential Human Reproductive and Developmental Effects of Di(2-ethylhexyl) Phthalate (DEHP)," draft, May 2006, http://cerhr.niehs.nih.gov/chemicals/dehp/DEHP%20Brief%20Draft1.pdf.

36. E.O. Dillingham and J. Autian, "Teratogenicity, Mutagenicity, and Cellular Toxicity of Phthalate Esters" *Environmental Health Perspectives* 3 (1973): 81–89.

37. M. R. Parkhie, M. Webb, and M. A. Norcross, "Dimethoxyethyl Phthalate: Em-

bryopathy, Teratogenicity, Fetal Metabolism, and the Role of Zinc in the Rat," *Environmental Health Perspectives* 45 (1982): 89–97.

38. National Toxicology Program, Center for the Evaluation of Risks to Human Reproduction, "Thalidomide," http://cerhr.niehs.nih.gov/common/thalidomide.html.

39. Department of Health and Ageing, NICNAS, "Existing Chemical Hazard Assessment Report: Bis(2-methoxyethyl) Phthalate," June 2008, at www.nicnas.gov.au/publications/car/other/DMEP%20hazard%20assessment.pdf.

40. The study was also conducted by the NTP's predecessor, the National Cancer Institute Carcinogenicity Bioassay program, a mouthful of a name that is a reminder of how, historically, materials' toxicology programs have focused on cancer effects.

41. The International Agency for Research on Cancer (part of the World Health Organization) also listed DEHP as a "possible carcinogen following the 1982 U.S. National Toxicology Program studies." In 2000, however, the IARC revised its judgment saying that the rodent data were not relevant to people, so in its view DEHP was "not classifiable as a human carcinogen," a classification later adopted by the European Commission.

42. American Chemistry Council, "Questions and Answers," www.american chemistry.com/s_phthalate/sec.asp?CID=1762&DID=6479.

43. American Chemistry Council, "What the Precautionary Principle Is?" www .americanchemistry.com/s_phthalate/sec.asp?CID=1914&DID=7593.

44. Hugh Taylor, personal communication with author, March 2007.

45. Patricia Hunt, personal communication with author, March 2007. American Chemistry Council, "FAQs: The Safety of Baby Bottles, Nalgene Sports Bottles, and Food Containers Made with Polycarbonate Plastic," www.plastics info.org/s_plasticsinfo/sec_level2_faq.asp?CID=704&DID=2838.

46. Paul Foster, Chemical Heritage Foundation conference, March 2007.

47. For a list of these hospitals, see Health Care Without Harm's website at www .noharm.org/us/pvcDehp/hospitalsreducingpvc.

48. Shanna H. Swan, personal communication with author, March 2007, and Ted Schettler, personal communication with author, August 2008.

CHAPTER 6: THE PERSISTENT AND PERNICIOUS

1. Division of Spell Prevention and Response, Contaminated Site Progrm, "St. Lawrence Island," October 2008, www.dec.state.ak.us/spar/csp/sites/stlawrence.htm.

2. Mirex, also known as dechlorane, is one of the dozen contaminants subject

to restriction under the Stockholm Convention on persistent organic pollutants.

3. Alaska Department of Environmental Conservation Contaminated Sites
   Database, "Cleanup Chronology Report for St. Law NEC Facility Wide," www
   .dec.state.ak.us/spar/csp/search/IC_Tracking/Site_Report.aspx?Hazard_ID
   =207.

4. D. O. Carpenter, A. P. DeCaprio, D. O'Hehir, F. Akhtar, G. Johnson, R. J.
   Scrudato, L. Apatiki, et al., "Polychlorinated Biphenyls in Serum of the Siber-
   ian Yupik People from St. Lawrence Island, Alaska," *International Journal of Circumpolar Health* 64, no. 4 (2005): 322–35.

5. Olivier Humblet, Linda Birnbaum, Eric Rimm, Murray A. Mittelman, and
   Russ Hauser, "Dioxins and Cardiovascular Disease Mortality," *Environmental
   Health Perspectives* 116, no. 11 (2008): 1443–48.

6. U.S. EPA National Center for Environmental Assessment, "Dioxin," June 29,
   2007, http://cfpub.epa.gov/ncea/CFM/nceaQFind.cfm?keyword=Dioxin. ·

7. U.S. Department of Health and Human Services et al., "Questions and Answers about Dioxins," January 2003, www.cfsan.fda.gov/~lrd/dioxinqa.html.

8. Linda S. Birnbaum, presentation at Dioxin 2007 conference, Tokyo, Japan, September 2007.

9. U.S. EPA Persistent Bioaccumulative and Toxic (PBT) Pollutant Chemical
   Program, "Dioxins and Furans," January 15, 2008, www.epa.gov/pbt/pubs/
   dioxins.htm.

10. Linda S. Birnbaum and Daniele F. Staskal, "Brominated Flame Retardants:
    Cause for Concern?" *Environmental Health Perspectives* 112, no.1 (2004): 9–17.

11. Ronald A. Hites, "Polybrominated Diphenyl Ethers in the Environment and
    People: A Meta-Analysis of Concentrations," *Environmental Science & Technol-
    ogy* 38, no. 4 (2004): 945–56.

12. Bromine Science and Environment Forum, "Human Health Research," Au-
    gust 2008, www.bsef.com/env_health. (This website has since been changed
    and alternate information is now supplied at http://www.bsef.com/our-
    substances/deca-bde/scientific-studies, where organization now describes the
    risks posed by deca-BDE as "low and manageable," by TBBPA as "no risk" to
    human health but toxic to aquatic organisms, and mentions no health or envi-
    ronmental impacts related to HBCD.)

13. Arnold Schecter, Dioxin 2007, Tokyo, September 2007.

14. U.S. EPA Integrated Risk Information System, "2,2',3,3',4,4',5,5',6,6'-Decabro-
    modiphenyl ether," July 1, 2008, www.epa.gov/iris/subst/0035.htm.

15. Adrian Covaci, Andreas C. Gerecke, Robin J. Law, Stefan Voorspoels, Martin Kohler, Norbert V. Heeb, Heather Leslie, et al., "Hexabromocyclododecanes (HBCDs) in the Environment and Humans: A Review," *Environmental Science & Technology* 40, no. 12 (2006): 3679–88.

16. Derek C. G. Muir and Phillip H. Howard, "Are There Other Persistent Organic Pollutants? A Challenge for Environmental Chemists," *Environmental Science & Technology* 40, no. 23 (2006): 7157–66.

17. K. J. Fernie, J. Laird Shutt, R. J. Letcher, I. J. Ritchie, and D. M. Bird, "Environmentally Relevant Concentrations of DE-71 and HBCD Alter Eggshell Thickness and Reproductive Success of American Kestrels," *Environmental Science and Technology* 43, no. 6 (2009): 2124–30.

18. Birnbaum and Staskal, "Brominated Flame Retardants."

19. R. F. Cantón, A. A. Peijnenburg, R. L. Hoogenboom, A. H. Piersma, L. T. van der Ven, M. van den Berg, and M. Heneweer, "Subacute Effects of Hexabromocyclododecane (HBCD) on Hepatic Gene Expression Profiles in Rats," *Toxicological Applied Pharmacology* 231, no. 2 (2008): 267–72.

20. Kellyn Betts, "More Clues to HBCD Isomer Mystery," *Environmental Science & Technology* 39, no. 7 (2005): 146A–147A.

21. Birnbaum and Staskal, "Brominated Flame Retardants"; see also L. T. van der Ven, T. van de Kuil, A. Verhoef, C. M. Verwer, H. Lilienthal, P. E. Leonards, U. M. Schauer, et al., "Endocrine Effects of Tetrabromobisphenol-A (TBBPA) in Wistar Rats as Tested in a One-Generation Reproduction Study and a Subacute Toxicity Study," *Toxicology* 245, nos. 1–2 (2008): 76–89.

22. Janet Raloff, "Allergic to Computing?" *Science News*, www.sciencenews.org/view/generic/id/1704/title/Food_for_Thought__Allergic_to_computing%3F.

23. Chemtura, Material Data Safety Sheet, Firemaster 550, effective date June 20, 2006.

24. Alexander H. Tullo, "Resting Easier," *Chemical & Engineering News* 81, no. 46 (2003): 43–44,

25. San Francisco Estuary Institute, "Characterization of the Brominated Chemicals in a PentaBDE Replacement Mixture and Their Detection in Biosolids Collected from Two San Francisco Bay Area Wastewater Treatment Plants," poster available at www.sfei.org/rmp/posters/08BFR_Poster_klosterhaus_shrunk.pdf.

26. Kellyn Betts "New Flame Retardants Detected in Indoor and Outdoor Environments," *Environmental Science & Technology* 42, no. 18 (2008): 6778. Julia

Scott, "Fire Retardant Discovered in Wastewater Plants That Discharge into the Bay," *Oakland Tribune,* August 11, 2008. Heather M. Stapleton, Joseph G. Allen, Shannon M. Kelly, Alex Konstantinov, Susan Klosterhaus, Deborah Watkins, Michael D. McClean, and Thomas F. Webster, "Alternate and New Flame Retardants Detected in U.S. House Dust," *Environmental Science & Technology* 42, no. 18 (2008): 6910–16.

CHAPTER 7: OUT OF THE FRYING PAN

1. J. Peterson Myers is coauthor with Theo Colborn and Diane Dumanoski of *Our Stolen Future* (1996), a landmark book on endocrine disrupters. Comments by John Peterson Myers made at AAAS 2007 conference and Cain Research 2007 conference, Chemical Heritage Foundation.

2. U.S. EPA New Chemicals Program, "Is a Filing Necessary for My Chemical?" www.epa.gov/opptintr/newchems/pubs/whofiles.htm.

3. EPA Fact Sheet, "Emerging Contaminant, 1,4 Dioxane," April 2008.

4. REACH, "What Is Reach?" http://ec.europa.eu/environment/chemicals/reach/reach_intro.htm.

5. Comments by Derek Muir made at the AAAS 2008 conference.

6. U.S. EPA Science Advisory Board, "Perfluorooctanoic Acid Review Panel," www.epa.gov/sab/pdf/sab_06_006.pdf.

7. In a 2006 scientific review, the EPA has described one widely used PFC as a "likely carcinogen," but that review process is ongoing.

8. Kurunthachala M. Kannan, Emily Perrotta, and Nancy J. Thomas, "Association between Perfluorinated Compounds and Pathological Conditions in Southern Sea Otters," *Environmental Science & Technology* 40, no. 16 (2006): 4943–48.

9. Antonia M. Calafat, Lee-Yang Wong, Zsuzsanna Kuklenyik, John A. Reidy, and Larry L. Needham, "Polyfluoroalkyl Chemicals in the U.S. Population: Data from the National Health and Nutrition Examination Survey (NHANES) 2003–2004 and Comparisons with NHANES 1999–2000," *Environmental Health Perspectives* 115, no. 11 (2007): 1596–1602.

10. Benjamin J. Apelberg, Frank R. Witter, Julie B. Herbstman, Antonia M. Calafat, Rolf U. Halden, Larry L. Needham, and Lynn R. Goldman, "Cord Serum Concentrations of Perfluorooctane Sulfonate (PFOS) and Perfluorooctanoate (PFOA) in Relation to Weight and Size at Birth," *Environmental Health Perspectives* 115, no. 11 (2007): 1670–76.

11. Chunyuan Fei, Joseph K. McLaughlin, Loren Lipworth, and Jørn Olson, "Prenatal Exposure to Perfluorooctanoate (PFOA) and Perfluorooctanesulfonate

(PFOS) and Maternally Reported Developmental Milestones in Infancy," *Environmental Health Perspectives* 116, no. 10 (2008): 1391–95.

12. The EPA's 2006 Scientific Advisory Board report on PFOA found young children to have higher chemical levels than adults.

13. Rebecca Renner, "Is Arctic PFOA Contamination a 'Blast from the Past?' *Environmental Science & Technology*, January 4, 2006.

14. Rebecca Renner, "EPA Finds Record PFOS, PFOA Levels in Alabama Grazing Fields," *Environmental Science & Technology* 43, no. 5 (2009): 1245–46.

15. Minnesota Public Radio, "Toxic Traces: Timeline," http://news.minnesota .publicradio.org/projects/2005/02/toxictraces/timeline.shtml.

16. EIATRACK Environmental Intelligence Analysis, "EU Adopts Restrictions on Perfluorooctane Sulfonates (PFOS), Subject to Derogations; Perfluorooctanoic Acid (PFOA) Kept Under Review," March 27, 2007, www.eiatrack.org/r/1169.

17. U.S. EPA, "News Release: EPA Announces Substantial Decrease of PFOA," February 4, 2008.

18. Scott Finn, "Bush EPA Sets So-Called Safe Level of C8 in Drinking Water," West Virginia Public Broadcasting, January 15, 2009.

19. Environmental Working Group, "Credibility Gap: Toxic Chemicals in Food Packaging and DuPont's Greenwashing: New Food Packaging Chemicals: No Health Data," June 2008, www.ewg.org/node/26641.

20. Rebecca Renner, "PFOA in People," *Environmental Science & Technology* 41, no. 13 (2007): 4497–4500.

21. Renner, "PFOA in People."

22. As Scott Mabury—one of the world's experts on the environmental impacts of fluorine compounds—and his colleague Jessica C. D'Eon of the University of Toronto commented in a 2007 paper, "The issue of human exposure is increasingly complicated as several sources are likely involved, with relative contributions varying with lifestyle and location." Jessica C. D'Eon and Scott Mabury, "Production of Perfluorinated Carboxylic Acids (PFCAs) from the Biotransformation of Polyfluoroalkyl Phosphate Surfactants (PAPS): Exploring Routes of Human Contamination," *Environmental Science & Technology* 41, no. 13 (2007): 4799–4805.

23. Comments from Jennifer Keller's presentation at the AAAS 2008 conference.

24. Magali Houde, Trevor A. D. Bujas, Jeff Small, Randall S. Wells, Patricia A. Fair, Gregory D. Bossart, Keith R. Solomon, and Derek C. G. Muir, "Biomagnification of Perfluoroalkyl Compounds in the Bottlenose Dolphin (*Tursiops truncatus*) Food Web," *Environmental Science & Technology* 40, no. 13 (2006): 4138–44.

25. Comments from Jennifer Keller's presentation at the AAAS 2008 conference.

26. David Lazarus, "Carcinogen Worries Stick to Food Packaging," *Los Angeles Times,* July 20, 2008.

27. DuPont, "About PFOA," www2.dupont.com/PFOA2/en_US/about_pfoa/index.html.

28. 3M, "Human Health and the Environment," http://solutions.3m.com/wps/portal/3M/en_US/PFOS/PFOA/Information/Health-Environment.

29. Olga Nadeinko, personal communication with author, August 2008.

30. DuPont, "Frequently Asked Questions—DuPont Capstone," March 31, 2008.

31. DuPont, "Frequently Asked Questions—DuPont Capstone," March 31, 2008.

32. M.J.A. Dinglasan-Panlilio and S.A. Mabury, "Significant Residual Fluorinated Alcohols Present in Various Fluorinated Materials," *Environmental Science and Technology* 40, no. 5 (2006): 1447–53.

33. Comments by Terry Collins made at the Gordon Cain Conference, Chemical Heritage Foundation, March 23, 2007.

34. See DuPont's MSDS Central at http://msds.dupont.com/msds/Mediator, first accessed August 2008 and still available as of March 2009.

35. U.S. EPA, "Section 8(e) of TSCA," www.epa.gov/opptintr/tsca8e/index.htm.

36. See the Thermolon website, www.thermolon.com/.

37. Advertising for GreenPan with Thermalon sold via Amazon.com and Home Shopping Network, hsn.com, accessed most recently May 25, 2009. See www.amazon.com/Green-Pan-Set-Black-Aluminum/dp/B001D6MQM0/ref=sr_1_1?ie=UTF8&s=home-garden&qid=1243278752&sr=8-1 and http://kitchen-dining.hsn.com/greenpan-with-thermolon-technology-the-gourmet-set_p-3663839_xp.aspx.

38. See the website of the Shinwoo Trading Company, www.ebiz.co.jp/cgi-bin/out1.cgi?name=comp&value=idsw22.

39. Structure of Coating-Layer for Heat Cooker, Wipo Patent, www.freepatentsonline.com/WO2008010639.html.

40. Comments by Paul Anastas made at the Green Chemistry and Environmental Health Conference, University of California, Irvine, November 10, 2008.

CHAPTER 8: NANOTECHNOLOGY: PERILS AND PROMISE OF THE INFINITESIMAL

1. All of these products are included in the Woodrow Wilson Center's inventory of those that contain nanomaterials: www.nanotechproject.org/index.php?id=44&action=view. The novel is *Prey* by Michael Crichton (New York: HarperCollins, 2002).

2. National Nanotechnology Initiative, "FAQs: Nanotechnology," www.nano .gov/html/facts/faqs.html.

3. Comments by Vicki Colvin made at the AAAS Conference, February 16, 2007.

4. Rhitu Chatterjee, "Calculating the Costs of Nanohazard Testing," *Environmental Science & Technology*, March 25, 2009.

5. The list contains more than 800 entries as of April, 2009: www.nanotech project.org/inventories.

6. Author's interview with Barbara Kern, June 7, 2007.

7. Author's interview with James Hutchinson, May 17, 2007.

8. Author's interview with Kristen Kulinowski, June 12, 2007.

9. For more information see the ICON homepage, www.icon.rice.edu/index .cfm. Also see the Wilson Center Project on Emerging Nanotechnologies, www.nanotechproject.org/publications.

10. See the homepage for the International Alliance for NanoEHS Harmonization, http://nanoehsalliance.org.

11. Comments by James Hutchinson made at the Safer Nanotechnology Conference in March 2007.

12. Author's interview with Paul Anastas, April 30, 2007.

13. Author's interview with Terry Collins, May 7, 2007.

14. J. J. Wang, B. J. Sanderson, and H. Wang, "Cyto- and Genotoxicity of Ultrafine TiO_2 Particles in Cultured Human Lymphoblastoid Cells," *Mutation Research* 628, no. 2 (2007): 99–106. T. R. Pisanic, J. D. Blackwell, V. I. Shubayev, R. R. Fiñones, and S. Jin, "Nanotoxicity of Iron Oxide Nanoparticle Internalization in Growing Neurons," *Biomaterials* 28, no. 16 (2007): 2572–81. Li Zheng, Tracy Hulderman, Rebecca Salmen, Rebecca Chapmen, Stephen S. Leonard, Shih-Houng Young, Anna Shvedova, et al., "Cardiovascular Effects of Pulmonary Exposure to Single-Wall Carbon Nanotubes," *Environmental Health Perspectives* 115, no. 3, (2007): 377–82. Katharine Sanderson, "Migrating Nanotubes Add to Asbestos Concern," *Nature News*, March 31, 2009.

15. Matthew Cimitile, "Nanoparticles from Sunscreens Damage Microbes," *Environmental Health News*, March 24, 2003.

16. Zhonghua Tong, Marianne Bischoff, Loring Nies, Bruce Applegate, and Ronald F. Turco, "Impact of Fullerene (C60) on a Soil Microbial Community," *Environmental Science & Technology* 41, no. 8 (2007): 2985–91.

17. Author's interview with Peter Lichty, June 7, 2007.

18. Author's interview with Gordon Wozniak, May 31, 2007.

19. Comments by Vicki Colvin made at AAAS Conference in San Francisco, February 16, 2007.

20. Author's interview with Barbara Karn, June 2007.

21. Project on Emerging Nanotechnologies, "Experts Argue Nano Food-Additives Require New Oversight," www.nanotechproject.org/news/archive/7055.

22. Britt E. Erickson, "Nanotech Law for European Cosmetics," *Chemical and Engineering News* 87, no. 13 (2009).

23. Project on Emerging Nanotechnologies, "Nanotech and Synbio: Americans Don't Know What's Coming," www.nanotechproject.org/news/archive/synbio_poll.

CHAPTER 9: MATERIAL CONSEQUENCES: TOWARD A GREENING OF CHEMISTRY

1. Terry Collins, personal communication with author in January and May 2007, and from talks for the Oregon Environmental Council in January 2007, Chemical Heritage Foundation Gordon Cain Conference in March 2007, and from his interview with Moira Gunn on "Tech Nation" in March 2008.

2. Terry Collins, "The Journey to Safe Chemicals," *Pittsburgh Post-Gazette*, August 20, 2008.

3. See NatureWorks LLC, "Fact or Fiction?" www.natureworksllc.com/product-and-applications/fact%20or%20fiction.aspx.

4. CDC, NIOSH Alert, "Preventing Asthma and Death from Diisocyanate Exposure," 1996, DHHS (NIOSH) Publication No. 96–111, www.cdc.gov/NIOSH/asthma.html.

5. In September 2008, the U.S. Government Accountability Office (GAO) issued a statement saying that the EPA's so-called Integrated Risk Information System (IRIS) was at "serious risk of becoming obsolete." For example, some of the studies cited on the IRIS entry for phthalates were, at the time of this GAO report, more than fifty years old.

6. U.S. EPA High Production Volume Challenge, "OECD SIDS Manual Sections 3.4 and 3.5," www.epa.gov/HPV/pubs/general/sidsappb.htm.

7. Beginning in about 1996, the U.S. EPA began an effort to establish criteria and methods for determining what constitutes endocrine disruption. That effort is ongoing but as of April 2009 had yet to be fully launched. See www.epa.gov/endo/pubs/regaspects/index.htm for more information.

8. Comments by Michael Wilson made at the HPVIS meeting in Austin on December 13, 2006.

9. American Chemistry Council, "Registration, Evaluation, and Authorization of Chemicals (REACH)," www.americanchemistry.com/s_acc/sec_mediakits.asp?CID=344&DID=1180.

10. Joseph Pereira, "Protests Spur Stores to Seek Substitute for Vinyl in Toys," *Wall Street Journal*, February 12, 2008.

11. Nike, "Environment," www.nike.com/nikebiz/gc/r/fy04/docs/environment .pdf.

12. While use of organic cotton now amounts to but one-tenth of 1 percent of the world's cotton consumption, its ripple effects are significant, influencing the food supply chain and local food products as well as taking pesticide exposure and emissions out of cotton crop production—one of the world's most chemical-intensive. In 2006, Wal-Mart became the world's largest purchaser of organic cotton, surpassing Nike (the previous world-record holder) and joining other retail chains including H&M, Target, and Marks and Spencer as well as dozens of other companies that include textile manufacturers, clothing designers, and retailers

13. In 2007, Catherine Hunt was also leader of technology partnerships at Rohm and Haas; comments by Catherine Hunt made at the ACS Green Chemistry Conference in June 2007.

EPILOGUE: REDESIGNING THE FUTURE

1. For more information on PFCs and human fertility, see Chunyuan Fei, Joseph K. McLaughlin, Loren Lipworth, and Jørn Olsen, "Maternal Levels of Perfluorinatedchemicals and Subfecundity," *Human Reproduction* 1, no. 1 (2009): 1–6. See also N. Johansson, H. Viberg, A. Fredriksson, and P. Eriksson, "Neonatal Exposure to Deca-Bromnated Diphenyl Ether (PBDE 209) Causes Dose-Response Changes in Spontaneous Behaviour, Cholinergic Susceptibility in Adult Mice," *NeuroToxicology* 29 (2008): 911–19. S. Jobling, R. W. Burn, K. Thorpe, R. Williams, and C. Tyler. "Statistical Modeling Suggests That Anti-Androgens in Wastewater Treatment Works Effluents Are Contributing Causes of Widespread Sexual Disruption in Fish Living in English Rivers," *Environmental Health Perspectives* 117, no. 5 (2009). J. Hogaboam, A. Moore, and B. P. Lawrence. "The Aryl Hydrocarbon Receptor Affects Distinct Tissue Compartments during Ontogeny of the Immune System," *Toxicological Sciences* 102, no. 1 (2008): 160–70.

2. Geophysical Research Letters, Vol. 35, L03503, doi:10.1029/2007GL031572, 2008, http://www.arctic.noaa.gov/detect/ice-seaice.shtml

3. Comments made at the AGU annual meeting in December 2008.

4. Comments by Jerry Heindel made at the Green Chemistry and Environmental Health meeting at the University of California, Irvine, November 10, 2008.

5. Comments by Terry Collins made at the Green Chemistry and Environmental Health meeting at the University of California, Irvine, November 10, 2008.

6. U.S. EPA New Chemicals Program, "Is a Filing Necessary for My Chemical?" www.epa.gov/opptintr/newchems/pubs/whofiles.htm#exempt.

7. Comments by Lynn Goldman made at the Green Chemistry and Environmental Health meeting at the University of California, Irvine, November 10, 2008.

8. Comments by Paul Anastas made at the Green Chemistry and Environmental Health meeting at the University of California, Irvine, November 10, 2008.

9. The Chemical Abstracts Service (CAS) registry is the world's largest and, according to the ACS, most authoritative collection of disclosed chemical substance information; see www.cas.org/ for more information.

10. Comments by Paul Anastas made at the Green Chemistry and Environmental Health meeting at the University of California, Irvine, November 10, 2008.

11. Comments by Lynn Goldman made at the Green Chemistry and Environmental Health meeting at the University of California, Irvine, November 10, 2008.

12. Comments by Paul Anastas made at the Green Chemistry and Environmental Health meeting at the University of California, Irvine, November 10, 2008.

APPENDIX

1. Paul T. Anastas and John C. Warner, *Green Chemistry: Theory and Practice* (New York: Oxford University Press, 1998), 30–55. BeyondBenign, available online at www.beyondbenign.org/greenchemistry/greenchem.html, with assistance from Amy Cannon, May 2009.

2. Comments by Paul Anastas made at the Green Chemistry and Environmental Health meeting at the University of California, Irvine, November 10, 2008.

SELECT BIBLIOGRAPHY

Adibi, Jennifer J., Russ Hauser, Paige L. Williams, Robin M. Whyatt, Antonia M. Calafat, Heather Nelson, Robert Herrick, and Shanna H. Swan. "Maternal Urinary Metabolites of Di-(2-Ethylhexyl) Phthalate in Relation to the Timing of Labor in a U.S. Multicenter Pregnancy Cohort Study," *American Journal of Epidemiology* 169, no. 8 (2009): 1015–24.

Anastas, Paul, and John Warner. *Green Chemistry: Theory and Practice.* Oxford: Oxford University Press, 1998.

Apelberg, Benjamin J., Frank R. Witter, Julie B. Herbstman, Antonia M. Calafat, Rolf U. Halden, Larry L. Needham, and Lynn R. Goldman. "Cord Serum Concentrations of Perfluorooctane Sulfonate (PFOS) and Perfluorooctanoate (PFOA) in Relation to Weight and Size at Birth," *Environmental Health Perspectives* 115 (2007): 1670–76.

Arctic Monitoring and Assessment Programme (AMAP) and Arctic Council Action Plan to Eliminate Pollution of the Arctic (ACAP). "FACT SHEET: Brominated Flame Retardants in the Arctic," January 2005. www.amap.no/documents/index.cfm?dirsub=/Fact%20Sheets%20-%20ACAP (accessed April 27, 2009).

Australian Government Department of Health and Ageing-NICNAS. "Existing Chemical Hazard Assessment Report —Bis(2-methoxyethyl) Phthalate," June 2008. www.nicnas.gov.au/publications/car/other/DMEP%20hazard%20assessment.pdf (accessed April 27, 2009).

Betts, Kellyn. "More Clues to HBCD Isomer Mystery," *Environmental Science &*
Technology 39, no. 7 (2005): 146A–147A.

———. "New Flame Retardants Detected in Indoor and Outdoor Environments,"
Environmental Science & Technology 42, no. 18 (2008): 6778.

———. "Unwelcome Guest: PBDES in Indoor Dust," *Environmental Health Perspec-*
tives 116, no. 5 (2008). www.ehponline.org/members/2008/116-5/focus.html
(accessed April 27, 2009).

Birnbaum, Linda S., and Daniele F. Staskal. "Brominated Flame Retardants: Cause
for Concern?" *Environmental Health Perspectives* 112, no. 1 (2004): 9–17.

Blount, Benjamin C., Manori J. Silva, Samuel P. Caudill, Larry L. Needham, Jim L.
Pirkle, Eric J. Sampson, George W. Lucier, Richard J. Jackson, and John W.
Brock. "Levels of Seven Urinary Phthalate Metabolites in a Human Reference
Population," *Environmental Health Perspectives* 108, no. 10 (2000): 979–82.

Calafat, Antonia M., Zsuzsanna Kuklenyik, John A. Reidy, Samuel P. Caudill, John
Ekong, and Larry L. Needham. "Urinary Concentrations of Bisphenol A and 4-
Nonylphenol in a Human Reference Population," *Environmental Health Perspec-*
tives 113, no. 4 (2005): 391–95.

Calafat, Antonia M., Lee-Yang Wong, Zsuzsanna Kuklenyik, John A. Reidy, and
Larry L. Needham. "Polyfluoroalkyl Chemicals in the U.S. Population: Data
from the National Health and Nutrition Examination Survey (NHANES)
2003–2004 and Comparisons with NHANES 1999–2000," *Environmental Health*
Perspectives 115, no. 11 (2007): 1596–1602.

Canadian Broadcasting Corporation News. "Ottawa to Ban Baby Bottles Made
with Bisphenol A," April 18, 2008.

Canton, R. F., A. A. Peijnenburg, R. L. Hoogenboom, A. H. Piersma, L. T. van der
Ven, M. van den Berg, and M. Heneweer. "Subacute Effects of Hexabromocyclododecane (HBCD) on Hepatic Gene Expression Profiles in Rats," *Toxicologi-*
cal Applied Pharmacology 231, no. 2 (2008): 267–72.

Carson, Rachel. *Silent Spring*. Boston: Houghton Mifflin, 1962.

Chatterjee, Rhitu. "Calculating the Costs of Nanohazard Testing," *Environmental*
Science & Technology, March 25, 2009.

Cimitile, Matthew. "Nanoparticles from Sunscreens Damage Microbes," *Environ-*
mental Health News, March 24, 2009.

Colborn, Theo, Diane Dumanoski, and John Peterson Myers. *Our Stolen Future: Are*
We Threatening Our Fertility, Intelligence, and Survival? A Scientific Detective Story.
New York: Dutton, 1996.

Collins, Terrence J., and Chip Walter. "Little Green Molecules," *Scientific American*,
March 2006, pp. 84–90.

Collins, Terry. "The Journey to Safe Chemicals," *Pittsburgh Post-Gazette*, August 20, 2008.

Cone, Marla. *Silent Snow: The Slow Poisoning of the Arctic*. New York: Grove Press, 2005.

Cook, J. W., and E. C. Dodds. "Sex Hormones and Cancer-Producing Compounds," *Nature*, February 11, 1933, pp. 205–6.

Cook, J. W., E. C. Dodds, and C. L. Hewett. "A Synthetic Oetrus-Exciting Compound," *Nature*, January 14, 1933, pp. 56–57.

Cook, J. W., C. Hewett, and I. Hieger. "Coal Tar Constituents and Cancer," *Nature*, December 17, 1932, p. 996.

Covaci, Adrian, Andreas C. Gerecke, Robin J. Law, Stefan Voorspoels, Martin Kohler, Norbert V. Heeb, Heather Leslie, Collin R. Allchin, and Jacob de Boer. "Hexabromocyclododecanes (HBCDs) in the Environment and Humans: A Review," *Environmental Science & Technology* 40, no. 12 (2006): 3679–88.

Crutzen, Paul J. "Geology of Mankind," *Nature* 415, no. 3 (2002): 23.

D'Eon, Jessica C., and Scott Mabury. "Production of Perfluorinated Carboxylic Acids (PFCAs) from the Biotransformation of Polyfluoroalkyl Phosphate Surfactants (PAPS): Exploring Routes of Human Contamination," *Environmental Science & Technology* 41 (2007): 4799–4805.

Deutschle Tom, Rudolf Reiter, Werner Butte, B. Heinzow, T. Keck, and H. Riechelmann. "A Controlled Challenge Study on Di(2-ethylhexyl) Phthalate (DEHP) in House Dust and the Immune Response in Human Nasal Mucosa of Allergic Subjects," *Environmental Health Perspectives* 116, no. 11 (2008): 1487–93.

Dillingham, E. O., and J. Autian. "Teratogenicity, Mutagenicity, and Cellular Toxicity of Phthalate Esters," *Environmental Health Perspectives* 3 (1973): 81–89.

Dinglasan-Panlilio, M. J. A., and S. A. Mabury. "Significant Residual Fluorinated Alcohols Present in Various Fluorinated Materials," *Environmental Science & Technology* 40, no. 5 (2006): 1447–53.

Dodds, E. C., and Wilfrid Lawson. "Synthetic Oestrogenic Agents without the Phenanthrene Nucleus," *Nature*, June 13, 1936, p. 996.

Environmental Working Group. "Credibility Gap: Toxic Chemicals in Food Packaging and DuPont's Greenwashing: New Food Packaging Chemicals: No Health Data," June 2008.

Fei, Chunyuan, Joseph K. McLaughlin, Loren Lipworth, and Jørn Olsen. "Prenatal Exposure to Perfluorooctanoate (PFOA) and Perfluorooctancsulfonate (PFOS) and Maternally Reported Developmental Milestones in Infancy," *Environmental Health Perspectives* 116, no. 10 (2008): 1391–95.

Fernández, Marina, Maria Bianchi, Victoria Lux-Lantos, and Carlos Libertun.

"Neonatal Exposure to Bisphenol A Alters Reproductive Parameters and Gonadotropin Releasing Hormone Signaling in Female Rats." *Environmental Health Perspectives* 117, no. 5 (2009): 757–62.

Finn, Scott. "Bush EPA Sets So-Called Safe Level of C8 in Drinking Water," West Virginia Public Broadcasting, January 15, 2009.

Fung, Karen Y., Isaac N Luginaah, and Kevin M Gorey. "Generating Hypotheses in Sentinel High-Exposure Places" *Environmental Health Perspectives* 6, no. 18 (2007).

Geiser, Kenneth. *Materials Matter: Toward a Sustainable Materials Policy*. Cambridge, Mass.: MIT Press, 2001.

Geisz, Heidi N., Rebecca M. Dickhut, Michele A. Cochran, William R. Fraser, and Hugh W. Duklow. "Melting Glaciers: A Probable Source of DDT to the Antarctic Marine Ecosystem," *Environmental Science & Technology* 42, no. 11 (2008): 3958–62.

Gross, Frederick C., and Joe A. Colony. "The Ubiquitous Nature and Objectionable Characteristics of Phthalate Esters in Aerospace Technology," *Environmental Health Perspectives* 3 (1973): 37–48.

Gouin, Todd, and Frank Wania. "Time Trends of Arctic Contamination in Relation to Emission History and Chemical Persistence and Partitioning Properties," *Environmental Science and Technology* 41, no. 17 (2007): 5986–97.

Herzog, E., H. J. Byrne, A. Casey, M. Davoren, A.-G. Lenz, K. L. Maier, A. Duschl, and G. J. Oostingh. "SWCNT Suppress Inflammatory Mediator Responses in Human Lung Epithelium in Vitro," *Toxicology and Applied Pharmacology* 234, no. 3 (2009): 378–90.

Hileman, Bette. "Panel Ranks Risks of Common Phthalate Additional Research Underscores Concerns about DEHP That Were First Expressed in 2000 Report," *Chemical & Engineering News* 83, no. 46 (2005): 32–36.

Hites, Ronald A. "Polybrominated Diphenyl Ethers in the Environment and in People: A Meta-Analysis of Concentrations," *Environmental Science & Technology* 38, no. 4 (2004): 945–56.

Hogaboam, J., A. Moore, and B. P. Lawrence. "The Aryl Hydrocarbon Receptor Affects Distinct Tissue Compartments during Ontogeny of the Immune System," *Toxicological Sciences* 102, no. 1 (2007): 160–70.

Howdeshell, Kembra L., Paul H. Peterman, Barbara M. Judy, Julia A. Taylor, Carl E. Orazio, Rachel L. Ruhlen, Frederick S. vom Saal, and Wade V. Welshons. "Bisphenol A Is Released from Used Polycarbonate Animal Cages into Water at Room Temperature," *Environmental Health Perspectives* 111, no. 9 (2003): 1180–87.

Houde, Magali, Trevor A. D. Bujas, Jeff Small, Randall S. Wells, Patricia A. Fair, Gregory D. Bossart, Keith R. Solomon, and Derek C. G. Muir. "Biomagnification of Perfluoroalkyl Compounds in the Bottlenose Dolphin (*Tursiops truncatus*) Food Web," *Environmental Science and Technology* 40, no. 13 (2006): 4138–44.

Humblet, Olivier, Linda Birnbaum, Eric Rimm, Murray A. Mittleman, and Russ Hauser. "Dioxins and Cardiovascular Disease Mortality," *Environmental Health Perspectives* 116, no. 11 (2008): 1443–48.

Hutchings, Jennifer, Cathleen Geiger, Andrew Roberts, Jacqueline Richter-Menge, Martin Doble, Rene Forsberg, Katharine Giles, et al. "Role of Ice Dynamics in the Sea Ice Mass Balance," *Eos* 89, no. 50 (2008): 515–16.

Infante Peter, Stephen E. Petty, David H. Groth, Gerald Markowitz, and David Rosner. "Vinyl Chloride Propellant in Hair Spray and Angiosarcoma of the Liver among Hairdressers and Barbers: Case Reports," *International Journal of Occupational and Environmental Health* 15, no. 1 (2009): 36–42.

Jobling, S., R. W. Burn, K. Thorpe, R. Williams, and C. Tyler. "Statistical Modeling Suggests that Anti-Androgens in Wastewater Treatment Works Effluents Are Contributing Causes of Widespread Sexual Disruption in Fish Living in English Rivers," *Environmental Health Perspectives* 117, no. 5 (2009).

Jacobson, J. L., and S. W. Jacobson. "Intellectual Impairment in Children Exposed to Polychlorinated Biphenyls in Utero," *New England Journal of Medicine* 335, no. 11 (1996): 783–89.

Johansson, N., P. Eriksson, and H. Viberg. "Neonatal Exposure to PFOS and PFOA in Mice Results in Changes in Proteins Which Are Important for Neuronal Growth and Synaptogenesis in the Developing Brain," *Toxicological Sciences* 108, no. 2 (2009): 412–18.

Johansson N., H. Viberg, A. Fredriksson, and P. Eriksson. "Neonatal Exposure to Deca-Brominated Diphenyl Ether (PBDE 209) Causes Dose-Response Changes in Spontaneous Behaviour, Cholinergic Susceptibility in Adult Mice," *Neuro-Toxicology* 29, no. 6 (2008): 911–19.

Kannan, Kurunthachala M., Emily Perrotta, and Nancy J. Thomas. "Association between Perfluorinated Compounds and Pathological Conditions in Southern Sea Otters," *Environmental Science & Technology* 40, no. 16 (2006): 4943–48.

Kissinger, Meg. "U.S. Lawmakers Move to Ban BPA from Food, Beverage Containers," *Milwaukee Sentinel Journal*, March 13, 2009.

Krimsky, Sheldon. *Hormonal Chaos: The Scientific and Social Origins of the Environmental Endocrine Hypothesis*. Baltmore: Johns Hopkins University Press, 2000.

LaPensee, Elizabeth W., Traci R. Tuttle, Sejal R. Fox, and Nira Ben-Jonathan. "Bisphenol A at Low Nanomolar Doses Confers Chemoresistance in Estrogen Receptor-Alpha-Positive and Negative Breast Cancer Cells," *Environmental Health Perspectives* 117, no. 2 (2009): 175–80.

Larsson, Malin, Bernard Weiss, Staffan Janson, Jan Sundell, and Carl-Gustav Bornehag. "Associations between Indoor Environmental Factors and Parental-Reported Autistic Spectrum Disorders in Children 6–8 Years of Age," *NeuroToxicology*, forthcoming.

Layton, Lyndsey. "Studies on Chemical in Plastics Questioned," *Washington Post*, April 27, 2008.

Lazarus, David. "Carcinogen Worries Stick to Food Packaging," *Los Angeles Times*, July 30, 2008.

Li, Zheng, Tracy Hulderman, Rebecca Salmen, Rebecca Chapman, Stephen S. Leonard, Shih-Houng Young, Anna Shvedova, Michael I. Luster, and Petia P. Simeonova. "Cardiovascular Effects of Pulmonary Exposure to Single-Wall Carbon Nanotubes," *Environmental Health Perspectives* 115, no. 3 (2007): 377–82.

MacDonald, Elaine, and Sarah Rang. *Exposing Canada's Chemical Valley: An Investigation of Cumulative Air Pollution Emissions in Sarnia, Ontario Area.* Toronto: Ecojustice, 2007.

Macdonald, R. W., D. Mackay, Y.-F. Li, and B. Hickie. "How Will Global Climate Change Affect Risks from Long-Range Transport of Persistent Organic Pollutants?" *Human and Ecological Risk Assessment* 9, no. 3 (2003): 643–60.

Mahaffy, Paul R., David Beaty, Mark Anderson, Glen Aveni, Jeff Bada, Simon Clemett, Dave Des Marais, et al. "Science Priorities Related to the Organic Contamination of Martian Landers," unpublished white paper, posted November 2004 by the Mars Exploration Program Analysis Group (MEPAG) at http://mepag.jpl.nasa.gov/reports/index.html.

Malkan, Stacy. *Not Just a Pretty Face: The Ugly Side of the Beauty Industry.* British Columbia: New Society Publishers, 2007.

Markowitz, Gerald, and David Rosner. *Deceit and Denial: The Deadly Politics of Industrial Pollution.* Berkeley: University of California Press, 2002.

McKibben, Bill. *The End of Nature.* New York: Anchor Books, 1989.

Meeker, John D., Antonia M. Calafat, and Russ Hauser. "Di(2-ethylhexyl) Phthalate Metabolites May Alter Thyroid Hormone Levels in Men," *Environmental Health Perspectives* 115, no. 7 (2007): 1029–34.

Meyer, Torsten, and Frank Wania. "What Environmental Fate Processes Have the

Strongest Influence on a Completely Persistent Organic Chemical's Accumulation in the Arctic?" *Atmospheric Environment* 41, no. 13 (2007) 2757–67.

Minnesota Public Radio. "Toxic Traces: Timeline," http://news.minnesota.public radio.org/projects/2005/02/toxictraces/timeline.shtml (accessed April 27, 2009).

Mittelstaedt, Martin. "Sarnia's Emissions Affecting Health, Study Says," *Toronto Globe & Mail*, October 4, 2007.

———. "Tests Find Bisphenol A in Majority of Soft Drinks," *Toronto Globe & Mail*, March 5, 2009.

Muir, Derek C. G., and Phillip H. Howard, "Are There Other Persistent Organic Pollutants? A Challenge for Environmental Chemists," *Environmental Science & Technology* 41, no. 8 (2007): 3030.

Muir, Jennifer. "Industry Fights Effort to Ban Chemical in Baby Products,"*Orange County Register*, August 8, 2008.

Newbold, Retha R., "Prenatal Exposure to Diethylstilbestrol (DES)," *Fertility and Sterility*, 89, supp. 1 (2008): e55–c56.

Olewinski, W. J., G. Rapier, T. K. Slawecki, and H. Warner. "Investigation of Toxic Properties of Materials Used In Space Vehicles—Technical Documentary Report No. AMRL-TDR-63-99," December 1963, Biomedical Laboratory, Aerospace Medical Division, Air Force Systems Command, Wright-Patterson Air Force Base, Ohio, Prepared Under Contract No. AF-33(657)-8029, General Electric Company, Missile and Space Division, Philadelphia, Pa.

Parkhie, M. R., M. Webb, and M. A. Norcross. "Dimethoxyethyl Phthalate: Embryopathy, Teratogenicity, Fetal Metabolism, and the Role of Zinc in the Rat," *Environmental Health Perspectives* 45 (1982): 89–97.

Pereira, Joseph. "Protests Spur Stores to Seek Substitute for Vinyl in Toys," *Wall Street Journal*, February 12, 2008.

Pisanic T.R., J. D. Blackwell, V. I. Shubayev, R. R. Fiñones, and S. Jin. "Nanotoxicity of Iron Oxide Nanoparticle Internalization in Growing Neurons," *Biomaterials* 28, no. 16 (2007): 2572–81.

Pozo, Karla, Tom Harner, Frank Wania, Derek C. G. Muir, Kevin C. Jones, and Leonard A. Barrie. "Toward a Global Network for Persistent Organic Pollutants in Air: Results from the GAPS Study," *Environmental Science & Technology* 40, no. 16 (2006): 4867–73.

Raloff, Janet. "Allergic To Computing?" *Science News*. www.sciencenews.org/view/generic/id/1704/title/Food_for_Thought__Allergic_to_computing%3F.

Raun, A. P., and R. L. Preston. "History of Diethylstilbestrol Use in Cattle,"

Unpublished paper, American Society of Animal Science, 2002, www.asas.org/Bios/Raunhist.pdf.

Reddy, Christopher M., John J. Stegeman, and Mark E. Hahn, *Oceans and Human Health: Risks and Remedies from the Sea.* Boston: Elsevier, 2008.

Renner, Rebecca. "Is Arctic PFOA Contamination a 'Blast from the Past?'" *Environmental Science & Technology*, January 4, 2006.

———. "PFOA in People," *Environmental Science & Technology* 41, no. 13 (2007): 4497–4500.

———. "EPA Finds Record PFOS, PFOA Levels in Alabama Grazing Fields," *Environmental Science & Technology* 43, no. 5 (2009): 1245–46.

Sanderson, Katharine. "Migrating Nanotubes Add to Asbestos Concern," *Nature News*, March 31, 2009.

Sathyanarayana, Sheela, Catherine J. Karr, Paula Lozano, Elizabeth Brown, Antonia M. Calafat, Fan Liu, and Shanna H. Swan. "Baby Care Products: Possible Sources of Infant Phthalate Exposure," *Pediatrics* 121, no. 2 (2008): e260–e268.

Savinova, Tatiana, Vladimir Savinov, Lyudmila Stepanova, Sergey Kotelevtsev, Geir Wing Gabrielson, and Janneche Utne Skaare. "Biological Effects of POPs on Svalbard Glaucus Gull," Norwegian Ministry of the Environment. www.npolar.no/transeff/Effects/Glaucous_Gull/Gull-Akvaplan.htm (accessed April 27, 2009).

Scott, Julia. "Fire Retardant Discovered in Wastewater Plants That Discharge into the Bay," *Oakland Tribune*, August 11, 2008.

Silva, Manori J., John A. Reidy, James L. Preau, Jr., Larry L. Needham, and Antonia M. Calafat. "Oxidative Metabolites of Diisononyl Phthalate as Biomarkers for Human Exposure Assessment," *Environmental Health Perspectives* 114, no. 8 (2006): 1158–61.

Smith, Caroline, and Hugh S. Taylor. "Xenoestrogen Exposure Imprints Expression of Genes (Hoxa10) Required for Normal Uterine Development," *The FASEB Journal* 21 (2007): 239–46.

Stalhut, Richard W., Edwin van Wijngaarden, Timothy D. Dye, Stephen Cook, and Shanna H. Swan. "Concentrations of Urinary Phthalate Metabolites Are Associated with Increased Waist Circumference and Insulin Resistance in Adult U.S. Males," *Environmental Health Perspectives* 115, no. 6 (2007): 876–82.

Stapleton, Heather M., Joseph G. Allen, Shannon M. Kelly, Alex Konstantinov, Susan Klosterhaus, Deborah Watkins, Michael D. McClean, and Thomas F. Webster. "Alternate and New Brominated Flame Retardants Detected in U.S. House Dust," *Environmental Science & Technology* 42, no. 18 (2008): 6910–16.

Steward, Paul W., Edward Lonky, Jacqueline Reihman, James Pagano, Brooks B. Gump, and Thomas Darvill. "The Relationship between Prenatal PCB Exposure and Intelligence (IQ) in 9-Year-Old Children," *Environmental Health Perspectives* 116, no. 10 (2008): 1416–22.

Stiles, Lori. "UA Scientist Leads U.N. Team Drafting Plan for Sand, Dust Storm Warning System," University Communications, University of Arizona, November 20, 2007. http://uanews.org/node/17041 (accessed April 27, 2009).

Stockholm Convention on Persistent Organic Pollutants. http://chm.pops.int/Convention/tabid/54/language/enP-US/Default.aspx (accessed April 27, 2009).

Struck, Doug. "Dust Storms Overseas Carry Contaminants to U.S.," *Washington Post*, February 6, 2008.

Susiarjo M., T. J. Hassold, E. Freeman, and P. A. Hunt, "Bisphenol A Exposure in Utero Disrupts Early Oogenesis in the Mouse," *PLoS Genetics* 3, no. 1 (2007): e5.

Taylor, Julia A., Wade V. Welshons, and Frederick S. vom Saal. "No Effect of Route of Exposure (Oral; Subcutaneous Injection) on Plasma Bisphenol A throughout Twenty-Four Hours after Administration in Neonatal Female Mice," *Reproductive Toxicology* 25, no. 2 (2008): 169–76.

Thornton, Joe. *Pandora's Poison: Chlorine, Health, and a New Environmental Strategy.* Cambridge, Mass.: MIT Press, 2000.

Tierney, John. "Ten Things to Scratch from Your Worry List," *New York Times*, July 29, 2008.

Tong, Zhonghua, Marianne Bischoff, Loring Nies, Bruce Applegate, and Ronald F. Turco. "Impact of Fullerene (C60) on a Soil Microbial Community," *Environmental Science & Technology* 41, no. 8 (2007): 2985–91.

Tullo, Alexander H. "Resting Easier," *Chemical & Engineering News* 81, no. 46 (2003): 43–44.

U.S. Centers for Disease Control, "National Health and Nutrition Examination Survey (NHANES)," April 19, 2009. www.cdc.gov/exposurereport (accessed Aprl 27, 2009).

U.S. Environmental Protection Agency. "Risk Assessment for Toxic Air Pollutants: A Citizen's Guide," originally published as EPA 450/3-90-024, March 1991. www.epa.gov/ttn/atw/3_90_024.html (accessed April 27, 2009).

———. "High Production Volume (HPV) Challenge," www.epa.gov/HPV/ (accessed April 27, 2009).

———. "Contaminants in Great Lakes Sport Fish Fillets," April 19, 2009. www.epa.gov/glindicators/fishtoxics/sportfishb.html (accessed April 27, 2009).

U.S. National Oceanic and Atmospheric Administration. "A Near Real-Time Arctic Indicator Website—Ice-Sea Ice." www.arctic.noaa.gov / detect / ice-seaice.shtml (accessed April 27, 2009).

U.S. National Park Service. "Western Airborne Contaminants Assessment Project: The Fate, Transport, and Ecological Impacts of Airborne Contaminants in Western National Parks (USA)," January 2008.

U.S. National Snow and Ice Data Center. "Arctic Sea Ice News and Analysis." http://nsidc.org/arcticseaicenews/index.html (accessed April 27, 2009).

Van der Ven, L.T., T. Van de Kuil, A. Verhoef A, C. M. Verwer, H. Lilienthal, P. E. Leonards, U. M. Schauer, et al. "Endocrine Effects of Tetrabromobisphenol-A (TBBPA) in Wistar Rats as Tested in a One-Generation Reproduction Study and a Subacute Toxicity Study," *Toxicology* 12, no. 245 (2008): 76–89.

vom Saal, F. S., B. T. Akingbemi, S. M. Belcher, L. S. Birnbaum, D. A. Crain, M. Eriksen, F. Farabollini, et al. "Chapel Hill Bisphenol A Expert Panel Consensus Statement: Integration of Mechanisms, Effects in Animals, and Potential to Impact Human Health at Current Levels of Exposure," *Reproductive Toxicology* 24, no. 2 (2007): 131–38.

vom Saal, F. S., J. R. Kirkpatrick, and B. L. Coe. "Environmental Estrogens, Endocrine Disruption, and Obesity," in *Obesity: Epidemiology, Pathophysiology, and Prevention,* ed. Debasis Bagchi and Harry G. Preuss, 33–41. Boca Raton, Fla.: CRC Press, 2006.

Wang, J. J., B. J. Sanderson, and H. Wang. "Cyto- and Genotoxicity of Ultrafine TiO2 Particles in Cultured Human Lymphoblastoid Sells," *Mutation Research* 628, no. 2 (2007): 99–106.

Warner, John. "Guest Editorial: Asking the Right Questions," *Green Chemistry* 6 (2004): 27–28.

Wilson, Michael P., with Daniel A. Chia, and Bryan C. Ehlers. "Green Chemistry in California: A Framework for Leadership in Chemicals Policy and Innovation," University of California, California Policy Research Center, 2006.

Wilson, N. K., J. C. Chuang, C. Lyu, R. Menton, and M. K. Morgan. "Aggregate Exposures of Nine Preschool Children to Persistent Organic Pollutants at Day Care and at Home," *Journal of Exposure Analysis and Environmental Epidemiology* 13 (2003): 187–202.

Wilson, N. K., J. C. Chuang, M. K. Morgan, R. A. Lordo, and L. S. Sheldon. "An Observational Study of the Potential Exposures of Preschool Children to Pentachlorophenol, Bisphenol-A, and Nonylphenol at Home and Daycare," *Environmental Research* 103, no. 1 (2007): 9–20.

Weiss, Bernard. "Can Endocrine Disruptors Influence Neuroplasticity in the Aging Brain?" *NeuroToxicology* 28, no. 5 (2007): 938–50.

Wildbrett, G. "Diffusion of Phthalic Acid Esters from PVC Milk Tubing," *Environmental Health Perspectives* 3 (1973): 29–35.

Woodrow Wilson International Center for Scholars. "Project on Emerging Nanotechnologies." www.nanotechproject.org (accessed April 27, 2009).

Yergin, Daniel. *The Prize: The Epic Quest For Oil, Money, and Power*. New York: Simon and Schuster, 1991.

Young, Samantha. "California Lawmakers Weigh Ban on Chemical Found in Baby Bottles, although Danger Is in Dispute," Associated Press, August 10, 2008.

INDEX

Elizabeth Grossman is the author of *High Tech Trash: Digital Devices, Hidden Toxics, and Human Health*, *Watershed: The Undamming of America*, and *Adventuring Along the Lewis and Clark Trail*. Her writing has appeared in *Mother Jones*, *The Nation*, *Salon*, the *Washington Post*, and other publications. She lives in Portland, Oregon.

About Island Press

Since 1984, the nonprofit Island Press has been stimulating, shaping, and communicating the ideas that are essential for solving environmental problems worldwide. With more than 800 titles in print and some 40 new releases each year, we are the nation's leading publisher on environmental issues. We identify innovative thinkers and emerging trends in the environmental field. We work with world-renowned experts and authors to develop cross-disciplinary solutions to environmental challenges.

Island Press designs and implements coordinated book publication campaigns in order to communicate our critical messages in print, in person, and online using the latest technologies, programs, and the media. Our goal: to reach targeted audiences—scientists, policymakers, environmental advocates, the media, and concerned citizens—who can and will take action to protect the plants and animals that enrich our world, the ecosystems we need to survive, the water we drink, and the air we breathe.

Island Press gratefully acknowledges the support of its work by the Agua Fund, Inc., Annenberg Foundation, The Christensen Fund, The Nathan Cummings Foundation, The Geraldine R. Dodge Foundation, Doris Duke Charitable Foundation, The Educational Foundation of America, Betsy and Jesse Fink Foundation, The William and Flora Hewlett Foundation, The Kendeda Fund, The Andrew W. Mellon Foundation, The Curtis and Edith Munson Foundation, Oak Foundation, The Overbrook Foundation, the David and Lucile Packard Foundation, The Summit Fund of Washington, Trust for Architectural Easements, Wallace Global Fund, The Winslow Foundation, and other generous donors.

The opinions expressed in this book are those of the author(s) and do not necessarily reflect the views of our donors.